Bernhard Pommer

Minimally Invasive Sinus Membrane Elevation

Bernhard Pommer

Minimally Invasive Sinus Membrane Elevation

for Maxillary Bone Augmentation

Südwestdeutscher Verlag für Hochschulschriften

Impressum / Imprint
Bibliografische Information der Deutschen Nationalbibliothek: Die Deutsche Nationalbibliothek verzeichnet diese Publikation in der Deutschen Nationalbibliografie; detaillierte bibliografische Daten sind im Internet über http://dnb.d-nb.de abrufbar.
Alle in diesem Buch genannten Marken und Produktnamen unterliegen warenzeichen-, marken- oder patentrechtlichem Schutz bzw. sind Warenzeichen oder eingetragene Warenzeichen der jeweiligen Inhaber. Die Wiedergabe von Marken, Produktnamen, Gebrauchsnamen, Handelsnamen, Warenbezeichnungen u.s.w. in diesem Werk berechtigt auch ohne besondere Kennzeichnung nicht zu der Annahme, dass solche Namen im Sinne der Warenzeichen- und Markenschutzgesetzgebung als frei zu betrachten wären und daher von jedermann benutzt werden dürften.

Bibliographic information published by the Deutsche Nationalbibliothek: The Deutsche Nationalbibliothek lists this publication in the Deutsche Nationalbibliografie; detailed bibliographic data are available in the Internet at http://dnb.d-nb.de.
Any brand names and product names mentioned in this book are subject to trademark, brand or patent protection and are trademarks or registered trademarks of their respective holders. The use of brand names, product names, common names, trade names, product descriptions etc. even without a particular marking in this works is in no way to be construed to mean that such names may be regarded as unrestricted in respect of trademark and brand protection legislation and could thus be used by anyone.

Coverbild / Cover image: www.ingimage.com

Verlag / Publisher:
Südwestdeutscher Verlag für Hochschulschriften
ist ein Imprint der / is a trademark of
AV Akademikerverlag GmbH & Co. KG
Heinrich-Böcking-Str. 6-8, 66121 Saarbrücken, Deutschland / Germany
Email: info@svh-verlag.de

Herstellung: siehe letzte Seite /
Printed at: see last page
ISBN: 978-3-8381-3640-0

Zugl. / Approved by: Wien, MUW, Diss., 2012

Copyright © 2013 AV Akademikerverlag GmbH & Co. KG
Alle Rechte vorbehalten. / All rights reserved. Saarbrücken 2013

TABLE OF CONTENTS

ABSTRACT / ZUSAMMENFASSUNG 5

1. INTRODUCTION TO MAXILLARY BONE GRAFTING 7

    1.1. Structure 7
    1.2. Implant Treatment in the Atrophic Posterior Maxilla 8
    1.3. Maxillary Sinus Anatomy 9
    1.4. Maxillary Sinus Physiology 23
    1.5. Maxillary Sinus Floor Augmentation 32

2. PREOPERATIVE PLANNING PROCEDURE 36

    2.1. Background 36
    2.2. Gel-Pressure Technique – Material and Methods 37
    2.3. Gel-Pressure Technique – Study Results 41
    2.4. Discussion 44

3. TECHNIQUES OF TRANSCRESTAL OSTEOTOMY 48

    3.1. Background 48
    3.2. Clinical Comparison of Surgical Techniques – Material and Methods 48
    3.3. Clinical Comparison of Surgical Techniques – Study Results ... 51
    3.4. Discussion 52

4. BIOMECHANICS OF TRANSCRESTAL SINUS MEMBRANE ELEVATION 59

   4.1. Background 59
   4.2. Biomechanical Properties of the Maxillary Sinus Membrane – Material and Methods 66
   4.3. Biomechanical Properties of the Maxillary Sinus Membrane – Study Results 69
   4.4. Impact of Surgical Technique and Internal Sinus Anatomy – Material and Methods 70
   4.5. Impact of Surgical Technique and Internal Sinus Anatomy – Study Results 74
   4.6. Meta-Analysis of Maxillary Sinus Septa – Material and Methods 77
   4.7. Meta-Analysis of Maxillary Sinus Septa – Study Results 79
   4.8. Discussion 83

5. SIMULTANEOUS IMPLANT PLACEMENT AND PRIMARY IMPLANT STABILITY 91

   5.1. Background 91
   5.2. Primary Implant Stability – Material & Methods 92
   5.3. Primary Implant Stability – Study Results 96
   5.4. Discussion 98

6. BONE REGENERATION AND IMPACT ON SINUS
   PHYSIOLOGY 102

   6.1. Background 102
   6.2. Bone Regeneration – Material and Methods 103
   6.3. Bone Regeneration – Study Results 104
   6.4. Impact on Sinus Physiology – Material and Methods 105
   6.5. Impact on Sinus Physiology – Study Results 109
   6.6. Discussion 112

7. CONCLUSIONS 117

8. REFERENCES 120

ABSTRACT

Transcrestal elevation of the maxillary sinus membrane provides a minimally invasive treatment option to augment bone volume for dental implant placement in the edentulous posterior maxilla. The present thesis details on surgical as well as preoperative planning procedures of an innovative technique to elevate the sinus membrane using gel pressure. The influence of internal sinus anatomy and biomechanical properties of the maxillary sinus membrane on maximum membrane elevation height is studied in human cadaver experiments and computed tomography-based analyses. Maxillary sinus septa and primary stability of simultaneously placed implants are investigated. Clinical study results on methods of transcrestal osteotomy and bone regeneration following maxillary sinus floor augmentation are presented.

ZUSAMMENFASSUNG

Die transkrestale Elevation der Kieferhöhlenschleimhaut ermöglicht minimalinvasive Knochenaugmentation zur Impantatversorgung im zahnlosen posterioren Oberkiefer. Die vorliegende Dissertation behandelt chirurgische Durchführung sowie präoperative Planung einer innovativen Technik zur Membranelevation mittels Gel-Druck. Experimentelle Humanleichenstudien und computertomographische Analysen beleuchten den Einfluss der internen Kieferhöhlenanatomie und der biomechanischen Eigenschaften der Kieferhöhlenschleimhaut auf die maximale Höhe der Membranelevation. Kieferhöhlensepten sowie die Primärstabilität von simultanen Implantaten werden untersucht. Ergebnisse klinischer Studien über Methoden der transkrestalen Osteotomie und Knochenregeneration nach Sinusbodenaugmentation werden dargelegt.

1. INTRODUCTION TO MAXILLARY BONE GRAFTING

1.1. Structure

The structure of the present thesis reflects the main steps of minimally invasive transcrestal sinus membrane elevation for maxillary bone augmentation: preoperative planning procedures using computed tomographic scans (chapter 2), transcrestal osteotomy (chapter 3), transcrestal sinus membrane elevation (chapter 4), simultaneous implant placement (chapter 5) and postoperative bone graft regeneration (chapter 6).

The thesis presents original research data of following scientific publications:

- *"Mechanical properties of the Schneiderian membrane in vitro"* by Bernhard Pommer, Ewald Unger, Daniel Sütö, Niklas Hack and Georg Watzek (Pommer et al. 2009)
- *"Gel-pressure technique (GPT) for flapless transcrestal maxillary sinus floor elevation: a preliminary cadaveric study on a new surgical technique"* by Bernhard Pommer and Georg Watzek (Pommer & Watzek 2009)
- *"Effect of maxillary sinus floor augmentation on sinus membrane thickness in CT"* by Bernhard Pommer, Gabriella Dvorak, Philip Jesch, Richard Palmer, Georg Watzek and André Gahleitner (Pommer et al. 2012a)

- *"Prevalence, location and morphology of maxillary sinus septa: systematic review and meta-analysis"* by Bernhard Pommer, Christian Ulm, Martin Lorenzoni, Richard Palmer, Georg Watzek and Werner Zechner (Pommer et al. 2012b)
- *"Primary implant stability in the sinus floor of atrophic human cadaver maxillae: impact of residual ridge height, bone density and implant diameter"* by Bernhard Pommer, Markus Hof, Andrea Fädler, André Gahleitner, Georg Watzek and Georg Watzak (Pommer et al. 2012c)
- *"Maximum height of transcrestal maxillary sinus membrane elevation using osteotomes vs. liquid or gel pressure: computed tomography-based analyses"* by Bernhard Pommer, Ewald Unger, Andreas Schaller and Georg Watzek (Pommer et al. 2013a)
- *"Transcrestal osteotomy for minimally invasive sinus floor elevation: a prospective clinical trial comparing drill- vs. osteotome-mediated techniques"* by Bernhard Pommer, Ewald Unger and Georg Watzek (Pommer et al. 2013b)

1.2. Implant Treatment in the Atrophic Posterior Maxilla

Endosseous dental implants to replace the natural tooth provide a reliable basis for fixed and removable dentures (Stellingsma et al. 2004). Reduced alveolar bone height in the edentulous posterior maxilla due to post-extraction ridge resorption and maxillary sinus pneumatization represents a major limitation in the use of dental implants (Tawil & Younan 2003). Surgical treatment options to overcome this limitation comprise either supplementary bone augmentation procedures or the exclusive use of implants reduced in length (das Neves et al. 2006). The key advantage of placing short implants is the avoidance of invasive bone augmentation surgery associated with donor site morbidity, additional treatment duration and financial burden (Nedir et al. 2004), however, current literature is still controversial in regard to the reliability and indications of short dental implants. No increased early failure rates of short implants were observed down to a minimal length of 7 mm (Pommer et al. 2011). While horizontal defects are predominant in the anterior maxilla, the edentulous posterior maxilla presents with sufficient subantral bone width of 6 mm on average (Att et al. 2009) but residual alveolar ridge heights of less than 5 mm in 43% of cases (Lundgren et al. 1996). Maxillary sinus floor augmentation to date represents the most predictable possibility to enable implant placement in these cases of severe alveolar bone resorption and pneumatization of the maxillary sinus.

1.3. Maxillary Sinus Anatomy

The paired maxillary sinuses – pneumatic cavities of the facial skeleton – are the largest of the paranasal sinuses, which include the frontal, ethmoidal, and sphenoidal sinuses. Although descriptions and drawings are known from Leonardo da Vinci (1489), Nathaniel Highmore first described the clinical significance of the maxillary sinus, thus also known as "antrum of Highmore", in his treatise Corporis Humani Disquisito Anatomica in 1651 (Wendler 1986). Among primates, humans show the most extensive pneumatization of the facial skull. While pneumatized spaces can be seen in most mammals, birds, and reptiles, no sinus cavities are found in aquatic mammals (Lund 1988). No conclusive theory on the functional role of the paranasal sinuses has yet been established, with some authors arguing that they merely represent nonfunctional evolutionary remnants. Due to their inherent disadvantages, such as a marked susceptibility to chronic disease, it might reasonably be assumed that sinuses, if they did not serve any physiologic or anatomic function, would probably have been selected out and obliterated during the evolutionary history of humans (Gannon et al. 1997).

Theories on the physiologic function of the maxillary sinus include (Blanton & Biggs 1969): (a) weight reduction to maintain equipoise of the head: as maxillary sinus pneumatization reduces the skull weight by only 1% of the total, weight reduction may not be the main function; (b) protection of intracranial structures: the sinus architecture may be suited to act as a shock absorber and stress distributor to protect the skull base against trauma; (c) thermal insulation of vital parts: if an insulating mechanism to maintain cranial temperature is assumed, why do Africans have larger sinuses than Eskimos?; (d) humidification and warming of inhaled air: as it takes 50 breathing cycles to exchange the entire air volume of the sinus, conditioning of air cannot be a significant function; (e) secretion of mucus to moisten the nasal cavity: in contrast to the nose with its 100,000 submucosal glands, the sinuses have 100 glands at most; (f) increasing the area for olfaction: the sinus membrane is made up of nonolfactory epithelium; (g) imparting resonance to the voice: the physical properties of the sinuses make them poor resonators and maxillary sinus augmentation does not modify the spectral characteristics of the voice (Tepper et al. 2003); and (h) influence on facial growth and architecture: the architectural theory is far more likely in that the craniofacial shape has an important bearing on sinus growth and the maxillary sinus plays an important role in the formation of facial contours.

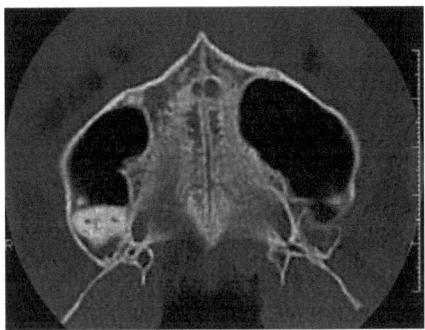

Figure 1.1: Axial computed tomography (CT) scan showing intra-individual variation of the size of the right and left maxillary sinuses.

The maxillary sinus shows significant anatomic variability. Its volume varies from 3.5 to 35 cm^3 with a mean size of 24 cm^3 in males and a significantly lower average of 16 cm^3 in females (Ariji et al. 1994, Uchida et al. 1998, Jun et al. 2005). The size of the maxillary sinus is significantly correlated with the external dimensions of the facial skeleton, while no differences are found between Angle's classes of skeletal malocclusion (Endo et al. 2010). Volume variations occur not only inter-individually, but also intra-individually, that is, bilaterally between the two sinuses of the same person (Figure 1.1). Forensic identification of skulls based on maxillary sinus analysis successfully predicts ethnicity in 90% and gender in 79% of cases (Fernandes 2004).

The maxillary sinus is a pyramidal cavity, with its quadrangular base forming the lateral wall of the nose and its apex extending into the zygoma. The roof of the sinus, which also constitutes the floor of the orbit, is composed of thin bone with the infraorbital neurovascular bundle in the central portion. The infraorbital canal is open towards the sinus in 14% of the population and thus in direct contact with the maxillary sinus membrane (Robinson & Wormald 2005). Its distal opening, the infraorbital foramen, can be found at a mean distance of 6.4 mm from the inferior orbital rim (Robinson & Wormald 2005) on the anterior (=buccal) wall, which corresponds to the canine fossa. The posterior (=infratemporal) wall separates the maxillary sinus from the pterygopalatine fossa and is formed by the maxillary tuberosity. The sinus floor is composed of the maxillary alveolar process and parts of the hard palate. It is normally located about 1 cm below the floor of the nasal fossa and may show alveolar recesses extending between adjacent teeth or roots of teeth (Figure 1.2).

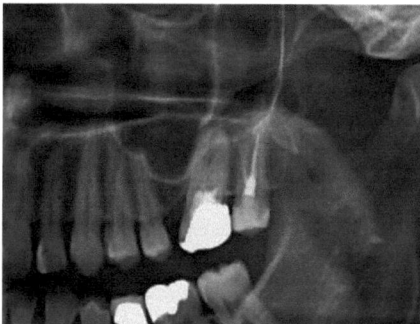

Figure 1.2: Alveolar recess of the maxillary sinus extending between adjacent teeth.

The maxillary sinus communicates with the ipsilateral nasal fossa through its natural orifice in the medial sinus wall, which also constitutes the lateral wall of the nose (Figure 1.3). The sinus ostium does not open directly into the nasal cavity, but into the floor of a narrow triangular space, the ethmoidal infundibulum. The infundibulum is demarcated by the uncinate process medially, by the lamina papyracea laterally, and by the ethmoidal bulla posteriorly. It communicates with the middle meatus of the nose through its nasal opening, the semilunar hiatus (Pignataro et al. 2008). The sinus ostium is a 7-11 mm long and 2-6 mm wide elliptical aperture with a mean surface area of 16.5 mm² (Xie et al. 2002, Pignataro et al. 2008). Usually found in the upper quarter of the medial sinus wall, it makes the drainage of the sinus inherently difficult anatomically. The diameter of the ostium is reduced on sitting up from a recumbent position (Aust & Drettner 1974). Accessory ostia have been found in 2% to 44% of individuals, anterior or posterior to the natural orifice, where the sinus is not separated from the nasal cavity by a bony component (Hood et al. 2009).

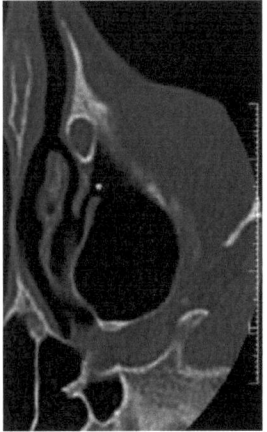

Figure 1.3: The medial sinus wall, which also constitutes the lateral wall of the nose, contains the natural sinus ostium (asterisk).

Average dimensions of the adult maxillary sinus are 35 × 25 × 32 mm vertically, transversely and anteroposteriorly (Woo & Le 2004, Flanagan 2005). The sinus floor is usually convex with its lowest point around the first and second upper molars (Figure 1.4). Its anterior border is located in the region of the second premolar (8%), the first premolar (58%) or the canine(33%), while its posterior border can be found in the third molar region in 94% of cases (Kim & Kim 2002).

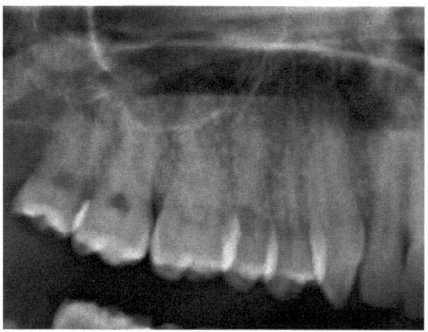

Figure 1.4: The lowest point of the maxillary sinus is usually found around the first or second maxillary molars with its anterior border in the region of the first premolar and its posterior border in the third molar region.

The maxillary sinus generally narrows as it approaches its anterior border in the premolar region. The angle formed by the inner buccal and palatal alveolar walls varies from 22 to 76 degrees (Figure 1.5) with a mean angulation of 36, 58, and 48 degrees at the second premolar, first molar and second molar sites, respectively (Velloso et al. 2006).

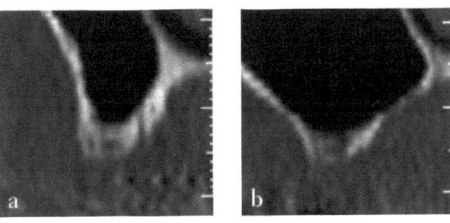

Figure 1.5: Comparison of narrow (a) and wide (b) angle formed by the inner buccal and palatal walls of the maxillary sinus.

While aplasia of the maxillary sinus is rarely encountered, sinus hypoplasia – defined as a horizontal or vertical size less than 50% of the corresponding orbital diameter – is seen in 5% to 10% of cases (Chrcanovic & Freire-Maia 2010). Despite the common view that infundibular obstruction may cause maxillary sinus underdevelopment, the majority of affected patients (70%, type I) present with moderate hypoplasia and a well-developed infundibular passage (Bolger et al. 1990), while 30% (type II + III) show a hypoplastic or absent uncinate process (Figure 1.6). Widening of the posterior ethmoidal cells into the maxillary sinus is known as "ethmomaxillary sinus". Present in 0.7% to 2% of people, it drains into the superior nasal meatus and is most frequently accompanied by a hypoplastic sinus (Selcuk et al. 2008).

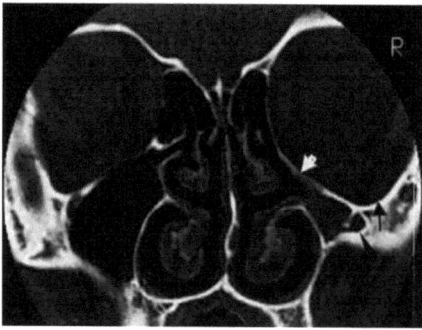

Figure 1.6: Maxillary sinus hypoplasia type III (as seen on the patient's right side) characterized by absence of the uncinate process (arrow) (Sirikçi et al. 2000).

Maxillary sinus hyperpneumatization is defined as a maximal horizontal or vertical size more than 90% of the corresponding orbital diameter (Kalavagunta &Reddy 2003). It is mostly bilateral with a prevalence of 8% and not necessarily associated with sinus pathology. Hyperpneumatization is termed "pneumatosinus dilatans" when it causes cosmetic impairment or local pressure symptoms and when the bony walls are intact (Lawson et al. 2008). When the bony walls are thinned or have lost their integrity, it is known as "pneumatocele" (Figure 1.7).

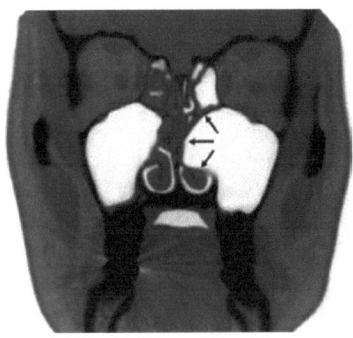

Figure 1.7: Pneumatocele of the maxillary sinus (Lawson et al. 2008).

Physiologic age-related sinus pneumatization is known as the fourth expansion phenomenon of the maxillary sinus and has been explained as a type of disuse atrophy. Posterior tooth loss has been shown to significantly support physiologic pneumatization and further reduce the bone mass due to crestal alveolar bone resorption. Progressive sinus pneumatization may also be due to metabolic processes, heredity, bone density, craniofacial configuration, positive sinus air pressure, and previous sinus surgery (Stübinger et al. 2010). According to Wolff's law a decrease of functional forces transferred to the bone after tooth loss causes a shift in the remodeling process towards bone resorption (Sharan & Madjar 2008). Histologically, the pneumatization process has been reported to be caused by increased osteoclastic activity in the sinus membrane, resorption of the cortical sinus floor, and deposition of osteoid inferior to it. As a result, the edentulous posterior maxillary alveolus consists of low-density trabecular bone with a minimal cortical layer and poor stress tolerance (Kim et al. 2006). In extreme cases of long-term edentulism, only a paper-thin bone plate separates the maxillary sinus from the oral cavity. Bone may have even been resorbed completely (Figure 1.8) so that the oral mucosa and the sinus membrane are in direct contact (Woo & Le 2004).

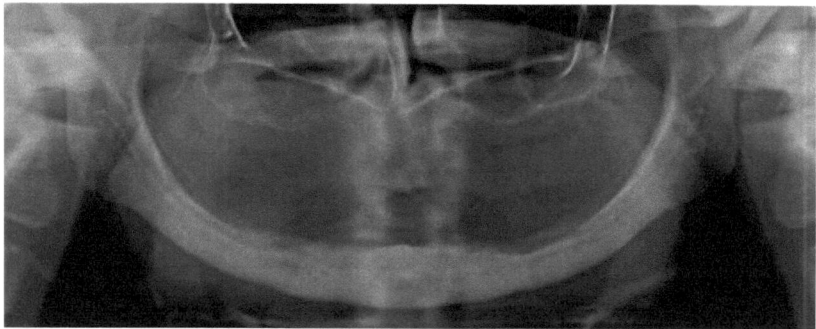

Figure 1.8: In long-term edentulism, only a paper-thin bone layer separates the maxillary sinus from the oral cavity.

The extent of sinus pneumatization varies both inter- and intra-individually. Post-extraction the maxillary sinus expands inferiorly by 1.8 mm, on average, within the first 5 years following tooth loss (Sharan & Madjar 2008). Significantly more extensive pneumatization occurs (a) after the extraction of teeth surrounded by a superiorly curving (concave) sinus floor (mean bone loss = 5.3 mm), (b) after second molar extractions compared with first molars, and (c) after the extraction of two or more adjacent teeth, while a residual anterior dentition appears to retard posterior bone resorption. Three subantral classes (SAC) of the edentulous upper posterior alveolar ridge have been distinguished (Nimigean et al. 2008): SAC 1 with a residual bone height of 10 mm (usually found in edentulism of no more than 5 years standing), SAC 2 with a residual bone height of 5-10 mm (after 5 to 10 years of edentulism, on average), and SAC 3 with a residual bone height of less than 5 mm (usually after edentulism of more than 10 years). It is obvious that bone height, along with low bone density, is the limiting factor for implant placement in the posterior maxilla, while the width of the alveolar crest ranges between 3.3 and 7.4 mm at molar sites even in extreme atrophy (Ulm et al. 1995).

The nerves supplying the maxillary sinus are derived from the maxillary division (V2) of the trigeminal nerve. The infra-orbital nerve (ION) is purely sensory and traverses the pterygopalatine fossa, where it gives off the posterior superior alveolar nerve (PSAN). The ION then enters the infraorbital canal, where it gives rise to the middle and anterior superior alveolar nerves (MSAN + ASAN) before emerging from the infraorbital foramen. The PSAN pierces the posterolateral sinus wall, courses between the bone and the sinus membrane (extraosseously) and forms a nerve plexus that supplies the maxillary sinus membrane (Murakami et al. 1994). By contrast, the MSAN and ASAN lie within the bony sinus wall (intraosseous) and form the superior dental plexus (Figure 1.9), which is located in the alveolar process (Graf & Martensson 1957); only a few branches of the PSAN join the plexus to innervate the maxillary teeth. Both the superior dental plexus and the plexus innervating the sinus membrane are present even in the absence of teeth (Robinson & Wormald 2005).

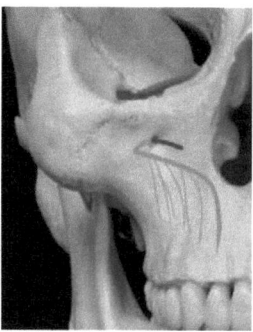

Figure 1.9: Schematic showing the intraosseous course of the anterior superior alveolar nerve, which contributes to the superior dental plexus.

Knowledge of the arterial supply of the maxillary sinus region is essential for surgical treatment and also has a bearing on the vascularization of sinus grafts (Elian et al. 2005). While the maxilla is densely vascularized in young and dentate individuals, the blood supply to the bone irreversibly reduces with age and progressive atrophy. Microvascular defects, stenoses, compromised intramedullary blood flow, suppressed osteoblastic activity, and delayed bone mineralization all result in a progressive loss of cancellous bone (Watzek et al. 1997). The periosteal blood supply, however, is maintained even after centro-medullary vessels have completely disappeared in severe maxillary atrophy (Solar et al. 1999).

The blood supply of the maxillary sinus is primarily derived from the posterior superior alveolar artery (PSAA) and the infraorbital artery(IOA), both branches of the maxillary artery (MA). In addition, the sphenopalatine artery supplies the inferior portion of the sinus. The PSAA branches off from the MA just as it enters the pterygopalatine fossa, and divides into one extraosseous and one intraosseous branch which enters the maxillary tuberosity (Flanagan 2005). The IOA accompanies the ION in the roof of the sinus (infraorbital canal), where it gives off the anterior (ASAA) and middle (MSAA) superior alveolar arteries. After emerging from the infraorbital foramen, the IOA supplies a terminal branch that forms an extraosseous anastomosis with the extraosseous branch of the PSAA (Figure 1.10) in 44% of individuals (Traxler et al. 1999). A second intraosseous anastomosis, also known as the alveolo-antral artery, is made with the other branch of the PSAA and the ASSA. It is seen in 100% of cases and is situated at a shorter distance from the alveolar ridge than the extraosseous one. The two anastomoses form a double arterial arcade supplying the lateral wall of the sinus and parts of the alveolar process (Rosano et al. 2010).

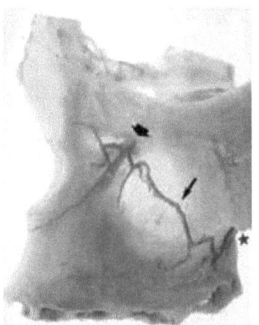

Figure 1.10: Extraosseous anastomosis (arrow) between the infraorbital artery (IA) and the posterior superior alveolar artery (asterisk) (Traxler et al. 1999).

The veins of the maxillary sinus empty into the facial vein and the pterygoid plexus (Dargaud et al. 2001), while the nasal sinus wall drains into the sphenopalatal vein (Chanavaz 1990). What is significant about the sinus venous drainage is that, apart from joining typical maxillary pathways to the jugular veins, it may also take an upward course to the cavernous sinus through the oval foramen (Figure 1.11) and the superior or inferior ophthalmic veins (Dazert et al. 2004).

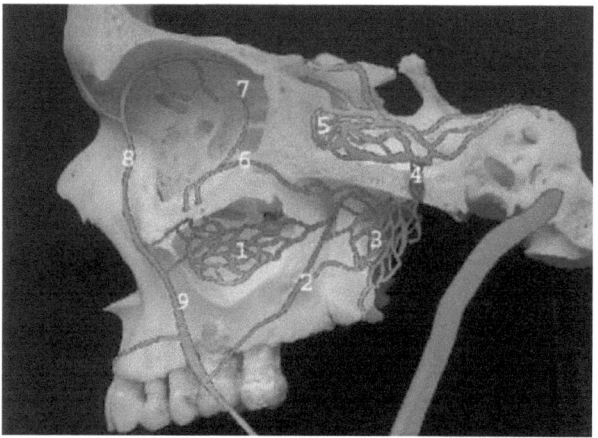

Figure 1.11: Venous connections of the maxillary sinus [1]: profound facial vein [2], pterygoid plexus [3], venous plexus of foramen ovale [4], cavernous sinus [5], inferior ophthalmic vein [6], anastomosis with superior ophthalmic vein [7], angular vein [8], facial vein [9] (Dazert et al. 2004).

From the cavernous sinus the blood flows into the deep middle cerebral vein, which communicates with the brain's superficial venous system through the white matter (Hauman et al. 2002). Spread of infection along this route is a serious complication of maxillary sinus infection (Figure

1.12). The lymphatic system of the maxillary sinus empties into collector lymph vessels within the mucosa of the medial nasal turbinate to reach the preauricular lymphatic plexus (Chanavaz 1990). In addition, lymph drains into the deep facial and deep cervical lymph nodes. Less well-known connections are to the auditory tube and the nasopharynx.

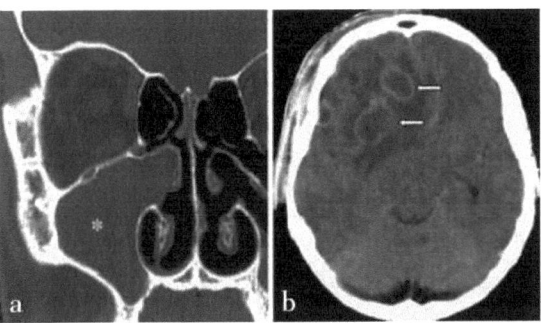

Figure 1.12: Spread of maxillary sinus infection (a) through the cavernous sinus into the endocranial compartment causing rhinogenic brain abscesses (b) (Dazert et al. 2004).

1.4. Maxillary Sinus Physiology

Along with mucociliary activity, the blood flow of the maxillary sinus mucosa is a key component of the defense mechanisms that serve to protect the maxillary sinus from infection. The sinus mucosa has a distinctly sparser vascular network than the nasal cavity, which is situated in the deepest layer of the lamina propria that rests on the periosteum (Flanagan 2005). However, blood flow to the maxillary sinus mucosa has been shown to be three times more abundant than that of exercised skeletal muscles

(Aust et al. 1978). Mucosal blood flow is regulated by the autonomic nervous system, and other factors such as gravity and endocrine activity also play a role (Falck et al. 1989). Vascular compromise may set in motion a series of events that predispose the antrum to the onset of sinus disease (Gannon et al. 1997).

Methods for a quantitative determination of the sinus mucosal blood flow in living patients include (1) plethysmography of the sinus membrane: manometry during ostium blockade and compression of the jugular veins (Drettner & Aust 1975); (2) xenon absorption by the sinus membrane: radioactivity uptake after inhaling ^{133}Xe during ostium blockade (Aust et al. 1978); and (3) laser Doppler velocimetry: endoscopy-guided perfusion flowmetry (Gannon et al. 1997). Blood flow and pulse amplitude in the maxillary sinus mucosa are considerably reduced during physical activity, falling to 44% of normal (Falck et al. 1989). Changes in posture from recumbent (0 degrees) to sitting (90 degrees) result in a decrease of the mucosal pulse amplitude of 0% (60 degrees), 5% (30 degrees), 14% (20 degrees) to a total of 21% (0 degrees), while the antral blood flow shows a decrease of 17%, 27%, 28%, and 35%, respectively (Falck et al. 1990a). Microcirculatory blood flow is also significantly reduced in patients with chronic sinusitis (Li et al. 2002). Decongestant nose drops have been found to strongly reduce mucosal pulse amplitudes and blood flow to the sinus mucosa while lowering the gas exchange in the mucosa by only a minor extent (Falck et al. 1990b).

Ventilation of the maxillary sinus is accomplished by gas exchange with the nasal cavity through the sinus ostium. Sinus ventilation may be quantified using xenon-enhanced CT techniques (inhalation of a xenon-oxygen-air mixture and repeated CT scans every 3 minutes) (Leopold et al.

2000). The mean washout time for a 95% exchange of sinus air is 5 to 20 minutes and shows extremely wide interand intra-individual variations (Hood et al. 2009). Both the size of the sinus ostium and the angle between the ostium and the nose affect the strength of the air stream and the amount of circulation (Müsebeck & Rosenberg 1978).

Air movement through the sinus ostium passes through four phases during one respiratory cycle. During inspiration the velocity of air rises to a peak in a very short time and then declines. The same two movements of air are observed in expiration, although the peak velocity is lower. The respiratory fluctuations in the nose induce a stream of circulation in the sinus. Differences in air velocity between the sinus and the nose are 1:50 to 1:100 and can be measured endoscopically by hot-film anemometry (Müsebeck & Rosenberg 1978). Maximal values of air velocity are recorded near the ostium, while minimal values can be found at the center of the sinus and the border of the zygomatic recess. Release of breathing stops the air movement in the sinus, while mucociliary action is not thought to influence sinus ventilation. Wider ostia and a shorter infundibular passage result in higher velocities and, therefore, are capable of higher transport rates (Hood et al. 2009). Air velocity in the sinus rises if the nasal mucosa contracts in response to decongestants. Three factors affect the efficiency of inhaled aerosolized particle deposition in the sinus: the size of the maxillary ostium, the pressure gradient, and the particle size of the aerosol. On topical aerosol delivery, particles smaller than 1 µm are more likely to reach the maxillary sinus, while larger particles appear to be deposited in the nasal vault (Hilton et al. 2008).

Under normal conditions, the temperature of the maxillary sinus is constant even when the external temperature changes (Perko 1991). An increased sinus temperature (higher than the body temperature) is seen in acute sinusitis, while chronic sinusitis, impaired sinus ventilation, or allergic conditions leave the temperature unchanged (Wodak 1961). Inspiration causes negative sinus pressure and expiration causes positive sinus pressure relative to the atmospheric pressure (Müsebeck & Rosenberg 1978). Sinuses with occluded ostia initially develop a positive pressure followed by negative pressure that reaches a subatmospheric plateau of –28.2 mm H_2O within 20 to 50 minutes (Scharf et al. 1995).

The gas exchange between the nose and the maxillary sinus is caused by fluctuations in breathing pressure and regulated by diffusion through the ostium (Müsebeck & Rosenberg 1978). Gas exchange in the sinus depends on (1) sinus volume, (2) size and shape of the nasal cavity, (3) the functional diameter of the ostium, (4) nasal airflow, (5) nasal respiratory pressure, (6) composition of gases, and (7) gas absorption by the sinus mucosa (Leopold et al. 2000). Compared with the atmospheric composition of air (78.1% N_2, 20.9% O_2, 0.03% CO_2), the gas composition in the sinus shows slightly supraphysiologic carbon dioxide levels (77.5% N_2, 18.8% O_2, 3.7% CO_2) (Mikula et al. 1996). An ostial diameter of less than 2.5 mm has been correlated with lowered oxygen and in creased carbon dioxide levels (Aust & Drettner 1974). Reduced oxygen tension has been shown to facilitate the growth of facultative anaerobic bacteria and to result in a marked reduction of mucociliary activity (Gannon et al. 1997). Compared with the nasal cavity, significantly higher concentrations of nitric oxide (NO) can be found in the sinus due to the presence of NO-synthase in the sinus mucosa (Kirihene et al. 2002). The low natural ventilation of the maxillary sinus may, in fact, be protective, as it not only prevents drying of the mucosal surfaces, but also helps to maintain a near-sterile environment with high NO concentrations and minimal pathogen access (Hood et al. 2009).

The bacteriology of the maxillary sinus under physiologic conditions has been widely investigated, however, the findings have been quite diverse. While healthy sinuses have traditionally been thought to be sterile, aerobic as well as anaerobic bacteria have been grown from 20% to 100% of asymptomatic sinuses. The most common aerobic isolates are B-hemolytic streptococci, staphylococci and Haemophilus sp., while counts of anaerobes routinely residing in the sinus, among them predominantly Bacteroides, Peptostreptococcus, and Fusobacterium sp., are lower (Brook 1981, Cook & Haber 1987). In contrast to the nasal mucosa which harbors a physiologic bacterial flora, it is still poorly understood whether these organisms represent normal habitants of the maxillary sinus or are transitory in nature. Some degree of inflammatory cell infiltration in the submucosa of the sinus membrane is considered normal for respiratory tissues. A host of specific and nonspecific defense mechanisms prevents maxillary sinus infection, i.e., mucociliary transport, neutrophils, macrophages, and the secretion of antimicrobial proteins and peptides by the maxillary sinus membrane (Carothers et al. 2001). The production of interleukin (IL)-1B stimulates the extravascular migration of polymorphonuclear neutrophils into the sinus (Tokushige et al. 1994). Human B defensins (HBD) exhibit broad-spectrum antimicrobial activity and may also act as chemoattractants for immature dendritic cells and T-cells, thus linking the innate and adaptive immune systems. Both HBD-1 and HBD-2 are present in the maxillary sinus mucus at concentrations of up to 130 ng/mL. A deficiency of these peptides may be a factor predisposing to chronic sinusitis (Carothers et al. 2001). In addition, NO produced by the sinus membrane is inhibitory to microorganisms, fungi, and viruses, and also stimulates mucociliary activity (Kirihene et al. 2002).

The maxillary sinus is lined by respiratory epithelium, which is represented by ciliated columnar cells, goblet cells, and basal cells resting on the basement membrane (Figure 1.13). The density of ciliated cells is very high, ranging from 91% to 98% except near the ostium (47%) (Guo et al. 1997). At the apical cell ends there are 100–150 cilia per columnar unit (Inanli et al. 2000), showing the characteristic 9 + 2 microtubular pattern (cylinder of nine pairs of microtubules encircling two single microtubules). Goblet cells and the openings of the submucosal glands are interspersed between the ciliated cells. Together these constitute the secretory elements of the sinus membrane. The goblet cells contain numerous mucin vesicles and have a mean density of 9,600 cells/mm^2 (compared with 5,600 cells/mm^2 in the nose) with wide individual variations, but no differences between the sinus walls (Toppozada & Talaat 1980). By contrast, the seromucous glands in the underlying stroma are scarce (mean density: 0.2 glands/mm^2) and predominantly located near the ostium. It must be assumed that the greater part of the mucus in the sinus is produced by goblet cells, while in the nose the greater part is produced by glands.

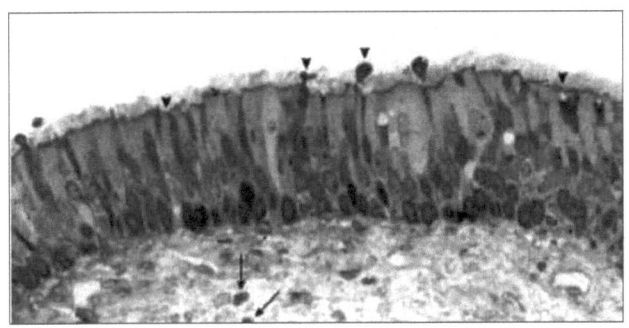

Figure 1.13: Light microscopy of the sinus membrane showing a pseudostratified ciliated epithelium with goblet cells (arrowheads) and a few inflammatory cells (arrows) in the submucosa (Timmenga et al. 2003).

The maxillary sinus mucosa is derived from the olfactory epithelium of the middle nasal meatus and thus shows great similarities to the epithelial ultrastructure of the nose, albeit with differences in fine details: the relatively diminished activity of seromucous glands, the delicate and loose epithelium, as well as the reduced number of cilia, indicate a lower resistance to infection and easier penetration of microorganisms (Toppozada & Talaat 1980). Diffuse mucosal thickening of the sinus membrane is found in up to 42% of subjects (Mathew et al. 2009). While mostly caused by odontogenic infections, i.e., periapical lesions and periodontal disease (58–78% of cases), mucosal thickening may also be associated with environmental allergy or upper respiratory tract disease and is not necessarily a sign of sinus infection (Kurien et al. 1989). Dentate subjects without dental pathology show the same prevalence as edentulous subjects (Vallo et al. 2010). Structural changes of the thickened sinus mucosa include edema, fibroplasia of the lamina propria, increased numbers of seromucous glands and goblet cells, interstitial cyst formation, and increased inflammatory cell infiltration (Toppozada & Talaat 1980).

The fundamentals of mucociliary clearance have largely been elucidated by Walter Messerklinger based on the observation that the human sinus mucosa and its ciliary activity survive 24 to 48 hours beyond the death of the individual (Pang et al. 2005). Mucociliary clearance eliminates both inhaled foreign bodies and hypersecreted respiratory mucus and depends on the complex interaction between motile cilia and mucus secretion (Toskala & Rautiainen 2005). The 2 L of mucus secreted per day consists of 96% water, 3–4% glycoproteins, immunoglobulins, lactoferrin, prostaglandins, lysozyme, leukotrienes, and histamine, and acts as an important immunological barrier (Pignataro et al. 2008). The maxillary sinus mucosa is covered by a double-layered mucous "blanket", which consists of the low-viscosity periciliary fluid and the highly viscous outer mucus (Asai et al. 2000). The cilia are in constant motion and act in concert to propel the overlying mucous blanket at a mean rate of 6 mm per minute (Tiwana et al. 2006).

Mucociliary transport runs along genetically determined stellate pathways originating from the sinus floor and ascending in a spiral to the natural ostium, even if alternative openings are created (Toppozada & Talaat 1980). The pattern of flow is specific for each individual sinus and seems to adapt to the inner sinus shape: by means of the so-called "bridging phenomenon", secretions thicken at rising bony edges and the gel phase slides over the serous phase in order to cross narrow passages (Pignataro et al. 2008). Occasionally, certain areas are noted to transport mucus faster than others. It is, however, not known whether these "secretion expressways" are artifacts caused by endoscopy (Pang et al. 2005). As the natural ostium is located in the upper quarter of the medial wall, secretion can only be removed by the active transport system of drainage and cannot take advantage of the force of gravity. Every 20 to 30 minutes the entire mucus of the maxillary sinus is renewed.

Rates of mucociliary clearance may be determined endoscopically using the saccharine time test, the India ink test (Asai et al. 2000), or by radioisotopic methods (Toskala & Rautiainen 2005). Effective mucociliary activity depends on multiple factors and requires a normal ciliary structure as well as normal ciliary function (Kim et al. 2008). Although the number of cilia, i.e., the ciliated area (percentage of mucosal surface occupied by cilia), may be normal, defective ciliary function may lead to impairment of mucociliary transport (Guo et al. 1997). The ciliary beat frequency (CBF) has been regarded as an indicator of effective ciliary movement, but even physiologic CBF values (10-20 Hz) do not guarantee proper mucociliary function (Abdel-Hak et al. 1998). The degree of variation in the beat direction of individual cilia, i.e., ciliary wave disorder (CWD), is another factor to be considered (Figure 1.14). Like a low CBF, high values of CWD may lead to impaired mucociliary clearance and consequent maxillary sinus pathology (Kim et al. 2008).

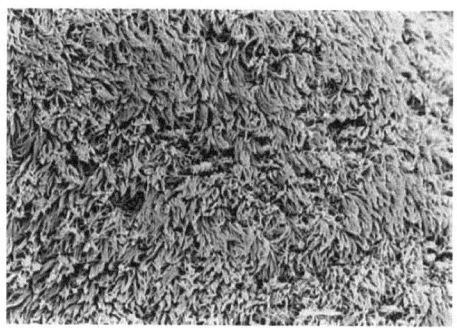

Figure 1.14: Scanning electron microscopy (magnification ×1000) of ciliary disorientation, resulting in impaired mucociliary transport (Asai et al. 2000).

1.5. Maxillary Sinus Floor Augmentation

The quantity and quality of available bone in the edentulous posterior maxilla is frequently compromised by pneumatization of the maxillary sinus cavity and postextraction alveolar bone resorption (van den Bergh et al. 2000, Ferrigno et al. 2006). Techniques for internal bone augmentation of the maxillary sinus floor have been established to permit reliable insertion of endosseous implants for prosthetic rehabilitation of this area. Internal augmentation of the maxillary sinus to compensate for sinus pneumatization is based on the principle of guided bone regeneration using the sinus membrane as a natural barrier. By coronal displacement of the maxillary sinus mucosa (Schneiderian membrane) with or either without addition of autologous bone or bone substitute material, the formation of vital bone to allow osseointegration of delayed or simultaneously placed implants is initiated (Berengo et al. 2004).

Membrane elevation is accomplished either via the lateral sinus wall (Figure 1.15), as described by Boyne in the 1960s, or via a transcrestal approach to the antrum, as decribed by Summers in the 1990s (Pjetursson et al. 2008). Systematic reviews on the survival of implants placed in the grafted maxillary sinus revealed average implant survival rates between 91.5% and 92.6% for the lateral approach, compared with survival rates between 93.5% and 96.4% for the transcrestal approach (Wallace & Forum 2003, Del Fabbro et al. 2004, Emmerich et al. 2005, Chiapasco et al. 2006). However, comparisons are difficult to be made, due to relevant differences in confounding variables, such as residual bone quantity and quality, grafting materials (or mixtures), implant geometry and surface, timing of implant placement and prosthetic loading, type of prosthesis and opposing arch dentition, patient-related factors, as well as implant success evaluation criteria (Chiapasco et al. 2006).

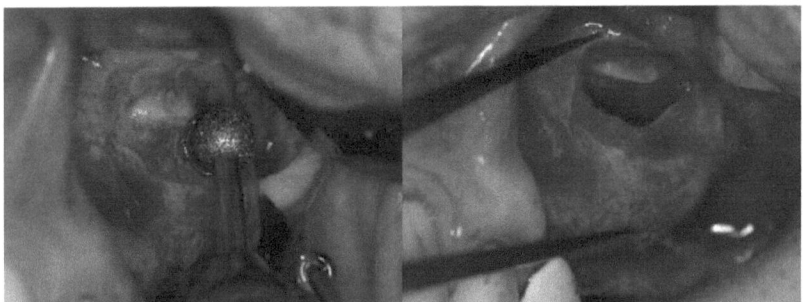

Figure 1.15: Sinus floor augmentation via a lateral approach (a) to gain sufficient bone height (b) for implant placement in the posterior maxilla.

The transcrestal approach to the maxillary sinus is advocated as 'minimally invasive' because of less postoperative morbidity and the undisturbed vascularization of the graft (Engelke et al. 2003). Besides the conventional osteotome-mediated transcrestal elevation (Summers 1994), various minimally invasive surgical techniques have been proposed: i.e. membrane elevation by inflation of a balloon catheter (Soltan & Smiler 2005, Kfir et al. 2006), the use of hydraulic pressure (Chen & Cha 2005, Sotirakis & Gonshor 2005, Vitkov et al. 2005), and negative pressure (Suguimoto et al. 2006).

The most common complication that occurs with all surgical techniques is the iatrogenic perforation of the Schneiderian membrane during elevation (Vlassis & Fugazzotto 1999, Ardekian et al. 2006). Membrane perforation rates have been reported to be 12–40% for the lateral approach (Khoury 1999, Mazor et al. 1999, De Leonardis & Pecora 2000). In transcrestal sinus elevation techniques perforation rates range between 2% and 25% (Berengo et al. 2004, Toffler 2004, Ferrigno et al. 2006). Perforation increases the chance of postoperative maxillary sinusitis due to bacterial graft contamination and/or graft migration into the sinus (Pikos 1999) and thus endangers graft as well as implant survival (Cho et al. 2001). Various options for managing these membrane tears during sinus augmentation via lateral antrostomy have been proposed, including closure with resorbable membranes (Mazor et al. 1999), fibrin adhesive (Sullivan et al. 1997), periostal patch (Nkenke et al. 2002), or resorbable sutures (Hernández-Alfaro et al. 2008). However, when transcrestal sinus augmentation techniques are applied, perforation of the Schneiderian membrane may not be recognized unless intraoperative antroscopy is carried out (Engelke & Deckwer 1997). Because of the limited access there is no possibility to repair the torn membrane without changing to a lateral surgical approach (Nkenke et al. 2002). Even in the absence of membrane perforations, postoperative sinusitis may occur at a mean rate of 3% and 1% following lateral and transcrestal augmentation, respectively (Pjetursson et al. 2008, Tan et al. 2008). Spread of infection to intracranial structures via the cavernous sinus is a rare yet serious complication. Total graft loss has been recorded at a mean rate of 2% in lateral sinus floor augmentation (Pjetursson et al. 2008).

2. PREOPERATIVE PLANNING PROCEDURE

2.1. Background

The transcrestal approach to the maxillary sinus is advocated as 'minimally invasive' because of less postoperative morbidity and the undisturbed vascularisation of the graft (Engelke et al. 2003). An important question concerning minimally invasive sinus augmentation is whether the obtainable amount of bone height is generally limited (Tepper et al. 2003, Engelke & Capobianco 2005) and therefore a conventional lateral approach should be preferred in cases of severely resorbed maxillae (Nkenke et al. 2002). The increase in bone height obtainable by osteotome-mediated transcrestal techniques has been shown to be inferior to that obtainable by the conventional lateral approach (Berengo et al. 2004). Another great concern in transcrestal sinus floor elevation techniques is the avoidance of iatrogenic sinus membrane perforation, as the elevation of the Schneiderian membrane is not performed under optical or tactile control (Toffler 2004). Due to the limited access there is no possibility to repair the torn membrane without changing to a lateral surgical approach (Nkenke et al. 2002).

Various modifications to the transcrestal osteotome-mediated sinus floor elevation technique have been reported in literature: membrane elevation by inflation of a balloon catheter (Soltan & Smiler 2005, Kfir et al. 2006), the use of hydraulic pressure (Chen & Cha 2005, Sotirakis & Gonshor 2005, Vitkov et al. 2005), or negative pressure (Suguimoto et al. 2006). The gel-pressure technique (GPT) was developed by o.Univ.Prof. DDr. Georg Watzek at the Department of Oral Surgery (Vienna Medical University, Austria) and represents a minimally invasive technique using a flapless surgical approach. As true for most surgical tactics that reduce invasion and duration of the intervention, as a result, the planning phase prior to surgery becomes more important and time-consuming.

2.2. Gel-Pressure Technique – Material and Methods

The aim of the following study was to introduce a new surgical technique for flapless transcrestal sinus floor elevation and evaluate the preoperative planning procedure in a human cadaver study (Pommer & Watzek 2009).

Edentulous maxillae of 4 fresh human cadavers (2 male and 2 female specimen, mean age: 73 years) were obtained from the Institute of Anatomy at Vienna Medical University, Austria. No formaldehyde fixation was carried out to avoid alteration in tissue consistency (Reiser et al. 2001). Immediately after preoperative CT scanning the maxillae were deep-frozen to -20° until prior to operation. Double-scan-technique CT scans were acquired with a conventional CT scanner (Tomoscan SR-6000, Philips, Eindhoven, The Netherlands) using a standard dental CT investigation protocol: 1.5 mm slice thickness, 1.0 mm table feed, 120 kV, 75 mA, 2 s scan time, 100-120 mm field of view, high-resolution bone filter (Gahleitner et al. 2003). Six radiopaque markers (gutta-percha balls) were placed into a polyvinyl siloxane impression of the edentulous jaw to perform the double-scan-technique (Verstrecken et al. 1996, Marchack & Moy 2003): the first scan was of the maxilla and the planning template in situ, the second of the planning template only. A computer assisted treatment planning software (Nobel Biocare, Yorba Linda, Calif.) allowed to superimpose the two sets of scans onto each other (van Steenberghe et al. 2002) and three-dimensionally plan the site of sinus trephination and implant position (Figure 2.1).

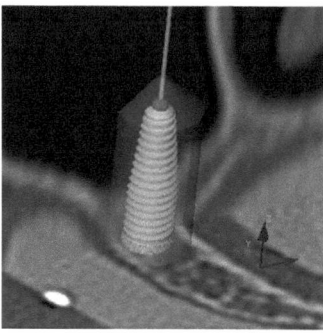

Figure 2.1: Presurgical three-dimensional planning procedure.

The planning data was transferred to a dental laboratory and a custom surgical template with precision titanium tubes was fabricated. The depth of the planned osteotomy was determined precisely in cross-sectional images at the elevation site (Figure 2.2) to facilitate puncture of the bony sinus floor without perforation of the adherent sinus membrane. The distance between the top edge of the planned implant and the bony sinus floor (value x) was measured in the center of the implant. The preplanned drilling depth was calculated by adding 10 mm to this value (9 mm distance between top edge of the planned implant and the top edge of the titanium tube, plus 1 mm height of the drill guide).

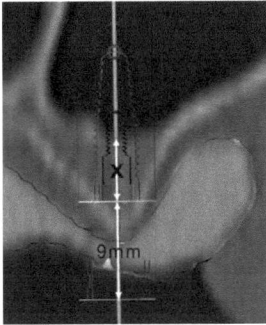

Figure 2.2: Measured distance x between the top edge of the planned implant and the bony sinus floor in the cross-sectional CT scan.

The surgical template was checked for proper seating and secured in place by 3 horizontal stabilization pins. A soft tissue punch of 4.1 mm diameter was carried out at the planned elevation site without mucoperiostal flap retraction. Cannon drills of 3.3 mm diameter (Friadent, Mannheim, Germany) with internal irrigation (Haider et al. 1993) were used for transcrestal osteotomies to puncture the bony floor of the sinus. Due to its rounded tip, this type of drill was considered more capable of preventing sinus membrane perforation than pointed drills. Custom-made drill depth stops were applied to reduce the length of the cannon drill to the preplanned drilling depth (Figure 2.3a). If no bony opening was created in the sinus floor by the first osteotomy, the drilling depth was increased by 0.5 mm (i.e. the height of the drill depth stop was decreased by 0.5 mm) until the bony sinus floor was punctured successfully. The integrity of the sinus mucosa was then evaluated by direct visual examination through the removed orbital floor. Thereafter a specially designed injection nozzle was inserted into the osteotomy and positioned 1 mm caudal to the bony sinus floor (Figure 2.3b). A silicon seal ring at the tip of the noozle was compressed by rotation of a screw nut to tightly obturate the osteotomy and secure the nozzle in place. Under controlled pressure a radiopaque gel was administered through the injection noozle to separate and elevate the Schneiderian membrane from the bony sinus floor until a total postoperative alveolar height of at least 15 mm was attained. Pressure control was achieved by a mechanical device attached to the injection noozle designed to limit the applied pressure to a maximum of 1 bar (100000 Pa) in all elevated sites.

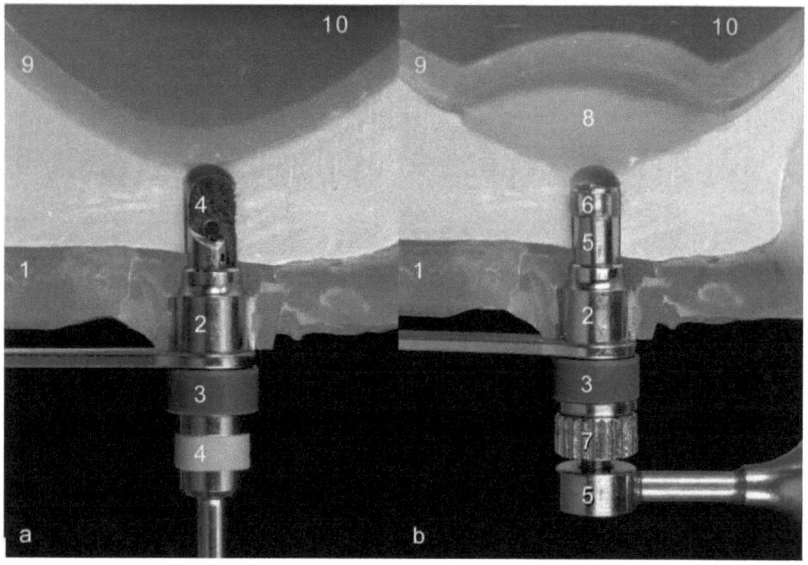

Figure 2.3: Procedure schematics. (a) guided transcrestal osteotomy. (b) gel injection. 1=surgical template, 2=drill guide, 3=drill depth stop, 4=cannon drill with internal irrigation, 5=injection nozzle, 6=silicon seal ring, 7=screw nut, 8=radiopaque gel, 9=Schneiderian membrane, 10=maxillary sinus.

Preoperative residual bone height, height of membrane elevation, and total postoperative height were assessed on postoperative CT scans and the amount of gel volume injected was recorded. Mean values are given with standard deviations. The integrity of the Schneiderian membrane was evaluated by direct visual examination through the removed orbital floor and on the postoperative CT scans. The Pearson's correlation coefficient (Williams 1996) was used to test following variables for linear relationship: Preoperative residual bone height was correlated to total postoperative height, preplanned drilling depth to actual drilling depth, and height of membrane elevation to gel volume injected. All calculations were done using R-project software (R Foundation for Statistical Computing, Vienna, Austria).

2.3. Gel-Pressure Technique – Study Results

A total of 10 flapless transcrestal sinus floor elevations were performed in 8 maxillary sinuses of 4 cadaver maxillae. The mean residual bone height of the alveolar crest was 4.7 ± 1.6 mm (range from 2.4 to 7.5 mm) at the elevation site (Table 2.1).

site	residual bone height (mm)	elevation height (mm)	total postop. height (mm)	gel volume (ml)	membrane perforation
16	2.4	12.6	15.0	3.1	no
26	6.9	8.4	15.3	1.1	no
16	4.6	10.6	15.2	2.1	no
25	6.2	8.6	14.8	2.0	no
26	4.4	10.7	15.1	2.1	no
27	3.9	11.4	15.3	2.3	no
16	7.5	8.0	15.5	0.9	no
25	2.8	12.1	14.9	2.8	no
16	4.5	11.2	15.7	2.2	no
26	3.3	11.9	15.2	2.7	no
total	4.7 ± 1.6	10.6 ± 1.6	15.2 ± 0.3	2.1 ± 0.7	0%

Table 2.1: Results of transcrestal sinus membrane elevation using the gel-pressure technique in 10 experimental sites.

Seating of the surgical template was satisfactory in all cases. To successfully puncture the bony floor of the maxillary sinus the preplanned drilling depth had to be increased by 0.5 mm in 1 site and by 1.0 mm in 3 sites. In the majority of cases (60 %) the planned drilling depth equaled the actual drilling depth showing a high statistical correlation (r=0.966). The bony opening created in the sinus floor was of smaller size than the diameter of the drill and no perforation of the Schneiderian membrane occured during the drilling procedure. The mean amount of gel volume injected was 2.1 ± 0.7 ml (range from 0.9 to 3.1 ml). The mean height of membrane elevation accounted 10.6 ± 1.6 mm (range from 8.0 to 12.6 mm). A strong statistical correlation between gel volume and height of elevation could be observed (r=0.929). Progressive gel injection resulted in circular, centrifugal dissection of the Schneiderian membrane and the formation of a dome-shaped subantral space (Figure 2.4a). In the left sinus of maxilla no.2 that was divided into 3 recesses by 2 bucco-palatal septa, each recess was sucessfully elevated without demonstrating a higher risk of membrane perforation (Figure 2.4b). The mean total height after membrane elevation amounted to 15.2 ± 0.3 mm (range from 14.8 to 15.7 mm). No statistical correlation between the residual bone height of the alveolar crest and the total postoperative height of the subantral space was found (r=0.320). In all tested sites, adequate elevation was attained to accommodate an implant of at least 13 mm length. No perforation of the sinus mucosa could be observed, neither by direct visual examination through the removed orbital floor, nor radiographically in postoperative CT scans (Figure 2.4c and 2.4d).

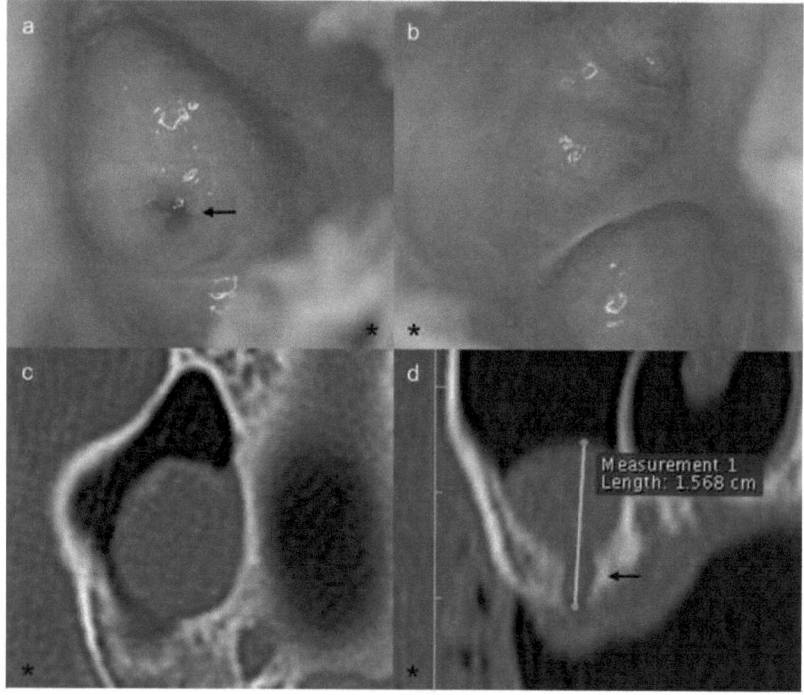

Figure 2.4: GPT-Membrane elevation in sinuses without (a) and with (b) sinus septa observed through the removed orbital floor. Postoperative axial (c) and cross-sectional (d) CT scans (arrow indicating the transcrestal osteotomy; * indicating the bucco-distal direction).

2.4. Discussion

Surgical techniques are of particular importance to increase the success rates of dental implants in the posterior maxilla (Nkenke et al. 2002). The new technique uses gel-pressure to elevate the maxillary sinus membrane for bone grafting of the bony sinus floor and simultaneous placement of endosseous implants using surgical templates. The method was modeled experimentally in fresh human cadaver maxillae. Intermediate freezing of the maxillae was necessary in order to preserve the cadaver tissues during the time required for fabrication of the surgical templates. Artefactual effects due to temerature alteration might be suspected in collagenous tissues. Studies revealed that relatively little protein denaturation occurs at –20°C (Bischof & He 2005) and cold denaturation of proteins is usually reversible in nature (Privalov 1990). No alteration in cell morphology after tissue sample storage was found with phase-contrast and dark-field light microscopy (Taylor et al. 1978). It may therefore be concluded that the surgical characteristics of the cadaver tissues were not significantly altered.

The main advantage of the gel-pressure technique (GPT) is the smooth transfer of force required for elevation of the maxillary sinus membrane from the bony underground. Compared to osteotome-mediated elevation techniques in which elevation forces are transferred to the sinus membrane via point transmission (Nkenke et al. 2002), the GPT allows for a bigger area of force transmission. By these means point forces that might exceed the elastic properties of the Schneiderian membrane are avoided. Sudden pressure that can cause sinus membrane perforation (Sotirakis & Gonshor 2005) is absorbed due to the cushioning effect of the highly viscous hydroxy-propyl-methylcellulose-gel used (4500 Pa). In the course of transcrestal sinus membrane elevation the force required for further membrane detachment increases along with the circumference of the created subantral space. Membrane perforation can occur as soon as elevation forces exceed the load limits of the Schneiderian membrane. Due to the optimized force transmission the height of membrane elevation obtainable with the gel-pressure technique may be superior to that obtainable with osteotome-mediated techniques. While intraoperative radiography during balloon-mediated membrane elevation at best confirms the integrity of the balloon itself, it reliably evaluates membrane integrity during the gel-pressure technique: if the sinus membrane is intact, a sharp contour is seen at the margins of the elevated area; if it is perforated, the contrast agent forms a fluid level in the sinus. On panoramic radiographs (with the patient standing) the fluid-level is seen in the horizontal plane. On CT scans (with the patient recumbent) it is seen in the frontal plane.

The gel-pressure technique represents a flapless transcrestal procedure to avoid exposure or removal of the lateral wall of the sinus. Advantages of the keyhole approach to the sinus include less alveolar resorption, better vascularization of the graft (Engelke & Capobianco 2005), minimal bleeding, less postoperative discomfort, and high patient acceptance. There is no intrinsic limitation of the technique if the initial bone height is severely reduced and secondary implant placement is required. In cases of maxillary septa, multiple transcrestal approaches can be chosen (Engelke & Deckwer 1997). The GPT combines the advantages of the lateral window approach, which permits the placement of high bone graft volumes, and the minimal invasivity of the transcrestal approach. Within the limits of a preliminary cadaveric study, it appears that the gel-pressure technique may be a practical method to correct alveolar deficiencies in the edentulous posterior maxilla. The height of sinus membrane elevation was not found to be limited and perforation of the Schneiderian membrane during elevation could be avoided. The results of the present study would suggest that this new surgical technique may reduce patient morbidity and extend the indication for transcrestal maxillary sinus floor elevation.

In minimally invasive sinus augmentation surgery both transcrestal osteotomy and maxillary sinus membrane elevation are performed without visual or tactile control (Toffler 2004). For this reason, precise three-dimensional planning is mandatory prior to grafting (Engelke & Capobianco 2005). Precise three-dimensional treatment planning is of particular importance in patients with knife-edge alveolar crests to avoid implant dehiscences that may go unnoticed due to the flapless surgical approach. This also applies to a narrow internal sinus anatomy, as buccopalatal deviations from the pre-planned implant alignment may make a significant difference for the desirable drilling depth (Figure 2.5).

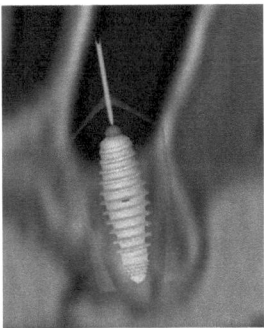

Figure 2.5: Pre-planned implant alignment in patients with a narrow sinus anatomy.

In less demanding cases the use of three-dimensional treatment planning software may not be necessary and a simpler, less time-consuming and more cost-effective approach may be chosen. For this approach a customized surgical stent with an integrated titanium tube is fabricated. The titanium tube helps to minimize radiologic artifacts. The stent is kept in place during the radiologic examination either by panoramic radiography or computed tomography.

3. TECHNIQUES OF TRANSCRESTAL OSTEOTOMY

3.1. Background

Transcrestal osteotomy to gain access to the maxillary sinus cavity is the first and most crucial operative step in minimally invasive sinus floor elevation surgery. The inherent difficulty that lies within this step is to predictably remove crestal alveolar bone in the absence of optical control without causing damage to the adjacent fragile maxillary sinus membrane (Pommer & Watzek 2009). Missing depth control may result in membrane perforation and thus abortion of the augmentation procedure at a very early stage (Stübinger et al. 2010). In one-stage sinus augmentation with simultaneous placement of dental implants, transcrestal osteotomy also constitutes bony preparation of the implant bed. Therefore, issues of potential thermal damages to collateral bone (Sasaki et al. 2002) as well as bone healing following osteotomy (Schwarz et al. 2007) need to be considered. Traditional techniques of transcrestal osteotomy involve the use of osteotomes or rotary devices (Kesler et al. 2006).

3.2. Clinical Comparison of Surgical Techniques – Material and Methods

The aim of the following study was to compare two surgical techniques of transcrestal maxillary sinus osteotomy, the use of osteotomes vs. drills, in a prospective clinical trial (Pommer et al. 2013b).

Twenty-five patients (13 men, 12 women, mean age of 45.6 ± 12.0 years) with deficient posterior maxillary ridges due to post-extraction sinus pneumatization were treated. A total of 34 sinuses (15 left sinuses, 19 right sinuses) were subjected to flapless transcrestal sinus floor elevation. Two different surgical techniques were used for transcrestal osteotomy to gain access to the maxillary sinus cavity: [A] osteotome technique: following the conventional osteotome-mediated transcrestal approach (Summers 1994) bone was removed up to 1 mm caudal to the sinus using drill stops and osteotomes were subsequently used to infracture the bony sinus floor (Figure 3.1), [B] drill puncture: transcrestal osteotomy was performed using drills with rounded tips and internal irrigation (Haider et al. 1993) to puncture the bony sinus floor without perforating the adjacent maxillary sinus membrane (Figure 3.2). Again drill stops of increasing height (0.5 mm difference between the drill stops) were used to precisely control the predetermined depth of the transcrestal osteotomy.

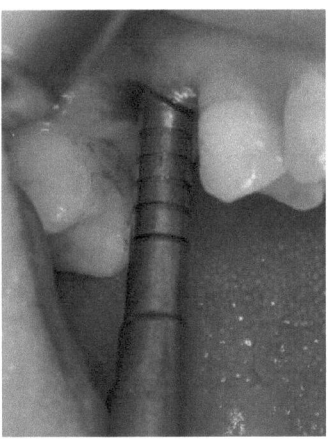

Figure 3.1: Transcrestal osteotomy by sinus floor infracture using osteotomes (group A).

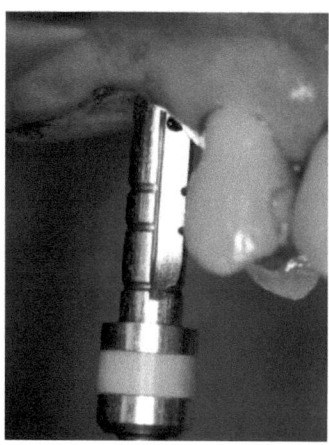

Figure 3.2: Transcrestal osteotomy using drills with rounded tips and internal irrigation (group B).

A radiopaque gel was injected into the transcrestal osteotomy to intraoperatively diagnose iatrogenic perforation of the maxillary sinus membrane using intraoral radiographs. The gel used consisted of 2% hydroxypropyl methyl cellulose (HPMC), a viscoelastic agent, and 37% iopamidol, a radiopaque marker, mixed at a ratio of 3:1 (Pommer & Watzek 2009). Purified trypan blue in a sterile 0.055% solution was added to the transparent gel to increase visibility intraoperatively (Agrawal et al. 2005). Hydroxypropyl methyl cellulose is a high-molecular-weight, water-soluble polymer, which is used in ophthalmic cataract surgery (Hosny et al. 2002) for gently opening the space needed for the procedure and protecting the tissues (Eisner 1983). A 2% HPMC solution is easily washed out (Chumbley et al. 1990), but does not cause a significant inflammatory response even when left behind and is no longer detectable after 3 days (Fleming et al. 1959, Smith et al. 1984, Liesegang et al. 1986). Likewise, iopamidol is an intravenous and gastrointestinal contrast agent which does not cause inflammatory tissue reactions of any kind (Ferrante et al. 1990).

Following transcrestal maxillary sinus membrane elevation using gel pressure and injection of bone substitute material (Pommer & Watzek 2009), a total of 40 implants (23 in male patients and 17 in female patients) were placed in a one-stage procedure. The mean implant length was 11.0 ± 1.4 mm (10 mm in 65% of cases and 13 mm in 35% of cases). The mean implant diameter was 4.3 ± 0.4 mm (3.5 mm in 15% of cases, 4.3 mm in 70% of cases and 5.0 mm in 15% of cases). The mean residual bone height of the atrophic ridges was 4.7 ± 1.8 mm. Preoperative bone height was at least 4 mm in 65% of cases. Maxillary sinus membrane perforation rate constituted the primary outcome measure and comparison between the two groups was performed using chi-square testing. Two sample t-tests were performed to compare residual alveolar ridge heights. The level of significance was set to $p<0.05$. All calculations were performed using R-project statistical software (R Foundation for Statistical Computing, Vienna, Austria).

3.3. Clinical Comparison of Surgical Techniques – Study Results

Of the 34 transcrestal sinus floor elevation surgeries included, transcrestal sinus osteotomy was performed using the osteotome technique in 17 procedures (group A, 50%) and in the other half of cases using drill puncture (group B, 50%). No significant difference regarding the residual alveolar ridge height in group A (5.1 ± 1.4 mm) vs. group B (4.5 ± 1.4 mm) could be found ($p=0.283$). Perforation of the sinus membrane was detected intra-operatively following sinus osteotomy in 2 cases using the osteotome technique (relative frequency of group A: 13%) and in 1 case using drill puncture (relative frequency of group B: 6%). The overall rate of maxillary sinus membrane perforation was 9% (Figure 3.3). No significant difference between the groups could be observed ($\chi^2=0.37$, p=0.544).

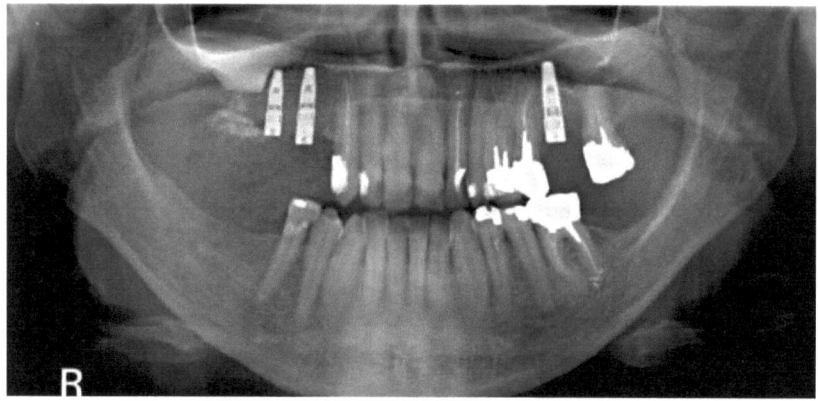

Figure 3.3: Radiographic evidence of maxillary sinus membrane perforation following transcrestal sinus osteotomy.

3.4. Discussion

Iatrogenic perforation of the maxillary sinus membrane may occur either during transcrestal osteotomy or in the course of membrane elevation. Only endoscopy reliably detects membrane tears (Engelke & Deckwer 1997), albeit at the cost of added invasiveness. The Valsalva procedure is indicative of membrane perforation only if positive (Ferrigno et al. 2006). A negative result, does, however, not confirm membrane integrity. Perforation may also be suspected, if the patient subjectively feels rinsing fluid in the nose. Exploring the elasticity of the membrane with a periodontal probe following transcrestal osteotomy (Cosci & Luccioli 2000) is unreliable and carries the risk of membrane perforation by probing. Contrast agents for imaging the maxillary sinus radiographically have been in use for over three decades (Sunukjian & DiFabio 1979) and represent a safer method to gain intraoperative evidence of iatrogenic membrane perforation following transcrestal sinus osteotomy.

On the one hand, the osteotome technique reduces the risk of iatrogenic damage to the maxillary sinus membrane due to system-inherent inaccuracy of preoperative planning using computed tomographies. The downside is, however, that infracturing the sinus floor may leave sharp edges on the mobilized bone segment, which are likely to increase the risk of membrane perforation in the course of subsequent maxillary sinus floor elevation. Clinical comparison of the 2 techniques showed no significant differences regarding rates of maxillary sinus membrane perforation between the groups. However, recent technological advances have led to increasing treatment options for dentoalveolar surgery, including piezoelectric surgery and laser devices (Romanos et al. 2009).

The use of piezoelectric surgery may provide a promising alternative to conventional techniques of transcrestal osteotomy (i.e. osteotomes or drills) to gain access to the maxillary sinus cavity. The ultrasonic frequency used in piezoelectric devices (29 kHz) is ideal for cutting mineralized tissue, but is ineffective in contact with soft tissue (Barone et al. 2008). In fact, a much higher frequency (50 Hz) would be needed to cut the latter (Schlee et al. 2006). Therefore, ultrasound technology may be used to overcome the precision and safety limits of conventional motor-powered instruments in oral bone surgery. The physical inability to cut soft tissue represents the most interesting surgical benefit of piezoelectric devices for maxillary sinus osteotomies. Furthermore, in-vivo experimental studies have shown increased rates of bone regeneration (Horton et al. 1975) and less damage to the adjacent bone at the structural and cellular levels (Vercellotti et al. 2005). No detrimental effects have been reported with regard to the viability and differentiation of cells growing out of autogenous bone grafts harvested from intraoral sites using piezoelectric devices (Chiriac et al. 2005).

The use of ultrasound curettes to carry out lateral-access osteotomies of the maxillary sinus was first proposed in 1998 (Torrella et al. 1998). Several clinical studies have investigated the risk of iatrogenic sinus membrane perforations associated with piezoelectric osteotomy. Reported membrane perforation rates are in the range of 5% to 30% (Vercellotti et al. 2001, Wallace et al. 2007, Barone et al. 2008, Stübinger et al. 2008). While some authors have postulated a reduced risk of membrane perforation using piezo-surgery (Vercellotti et al. 2001, Stübinger et al. 2008), the only randomized split-mouth study comparing piezoelectric devices with conventional rotating diamond-studded burrs showed no significant differences in the rate of membrane perforations (Barone et al. 2008). However, there is scientific evidence suggesting that, despite their cut selectivity, ultrasonic devices still carry a general risk of mechanically damaging the sinus membrane (Stübinger et al. 2005). While the pressure needed with the ultrasonic handpiece may be lower than that with rotating burrs, excessive mechanical forces from the instrument tip may still cause perforation of the sinus membrane (Schlee et al. 2006). This may be of particular relevance when leaving the compact bone and entering the less dense cancellous bone or the maxillary sinus.

The use of ultrasound technology has also been suggested in maxillary sinus osteotomies using a transcrestal approach (Figure 3.4). However, it is still poorly understood whether the lack of irrigation deep down in transcrestal osteotomy cavities causes thermal alterations in the hard and soft tissue structures (Stübinger et al. 2005). When the progress of the ultrasound tip is limited by too much pressure, heat is generated. Energy is also propagated to the soft and hard tissues as heat when the mechanical energy of the device is not used for cutting mineralized structures (Schlee et al. 2006). To date, there is no scientific evidence supporting the use of piezoelectric devices for facilitating maxillary sinus osteotomies carried out via transcrestal access.

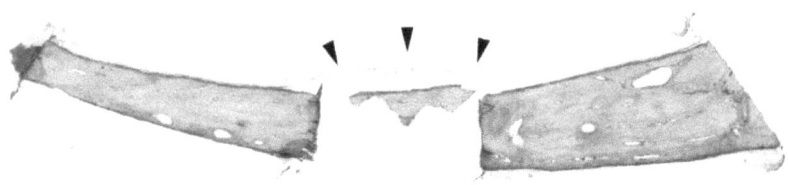

Figure 3.4: No evidence of maxillary sinus membrane perforation (arrows) following sinus osteotomy using a piezoelectric trephine.

Another treatment option for transcrestal osteotomy to puncture the bony sinus floor is laser technology. Laser devices were developed in the 1960s and their applications continue to expand in hard as well as soft tissue treatments in dentistry (Sohn et al. 2009). As burrs are among the most inconvenient and problematic tools in oral surgery for many patients, laser osteotomy could provide an elegant alternative (Deppe & Horch 2007). Histologically, erbium-doped yttrium aluminum garnet (Er:YAG) as well as erbium, chromium-doped yttrium scandium gallium garnet (Er,Cr:YSGG) laser irradiation has been found to cause less collateral bone damage than conventional drilling (Kesler et al. 2006), without signs of thermal side effects such as carbonization or melting (Kimura et al. 2001). Although present, minimal microstructural changes of the original apatites and reduction of the organic matrix are limited to a very thin area of 13–30 µm (Sasaki et al. 2002). These consist of numerous micro-cracks in the superficial layer, while the deep layer is less affected. CO_2 laser radiation, by contrast, causes extensive thermal side-effects up to a depth of 254 µm (Schwarz et al. 2007). This difference is most likely due to the optical characteristics of laser wavelengths, as Er:YAG and Er,Cr:YSGG lasers have a 10 times higher absorption coefficient of water than CO2 lasers (Schwarz et al. 2007).

Due to the lack of a smear layer and its characteristic irregular surface pattern, laser irradiation was assumed to potentially enhance the process of bone regeneration, i.e., the adhesion of blood elements. Comparative studies of titanium implant osseointegration showed faster initial bone healing following laser-assisted implant site development (Pourzarandian et al. 2004). Laser osteotomies frequently produce significantly wider peri-implant gaps particularly in the apical area, however, the percentage of bone-to-implant contact after 3 months of healing (64–73%) has been shown to be higher than, or equivalent to, conventional drilling (Kesler et al. 2006, Schwarz et al. 2007). These data at least seem to indicate that laser osteotomies do not compromise bone regeneration and the osseointegration of dental implants.

The first lateral sinus floor elevation using an Er:YAG laser was performed in 2002 (Jovanovic 2002). Since there is no need to exert pressure on the bone, laser osteotomies may be superior to mechanical drilling in terms of avoiding sinus membrane perforation. However, studies on the use of laser systems for lateral-access sinus osteotomies have reported membrane perforation rates of 33% to 100% (Table 3.1). While the applied laser parameters do not seem to be practicable for any clinical sinus elevation procedure (Stübinger et al. 2010), these investigations prove that laser osteotomies may cause perforation if they impinge on the sinus membrane.

study	laser	wavelength	pulse duration	frequency	perforation rate
Sohn et al. 2009	Er,Cr:YSGG	2.78 μm	140 μs	20 Hz	33%
Stübinger et al. 2010	Er:YAG	2.94 μm	300 μs	12 Hz	100%

Table 3.1: Summary of reported sinus membrane perforation rates in laser-assisted lateral sinus floor elevation procedures.

In transcrestal-access osteotomies of the maxillary sinus the use of lasers is still experimental (Deppe & Horch 2007). As the amount of bone removal per laser pulse is predetermined (0.66 mm cutting depth per Er:YAG pulse), the depth may be accurately gauged by using appropriate settings (Kesler et al. 2006). However, the depth of bone perforation has been found to be limited to 3 to 4 mm, as the efficiency of bone ablation is reduced by cancellous bleeding (Sohn et al. 2009). In addition, the bottom of the osteotomy cavity cannot be sufficiently cooled during laser irradiation. Currently, carrying out complete osteotomies in both length and diameter is not a workable prospect with any laser device (Romanos et al. 2009). It might be justified to develop quartz glass fiber tips adapted to the planned depth of the osteotomy for more homogeneous implant site development and for minimizing the risk of sinus membrane perforation (Schwarz et al. 2007). Further studies using various energy settings are needed to optimize the efficiency of laser osteotomies in transcrestal sinus floor elevation procedures (Figure 3.5).

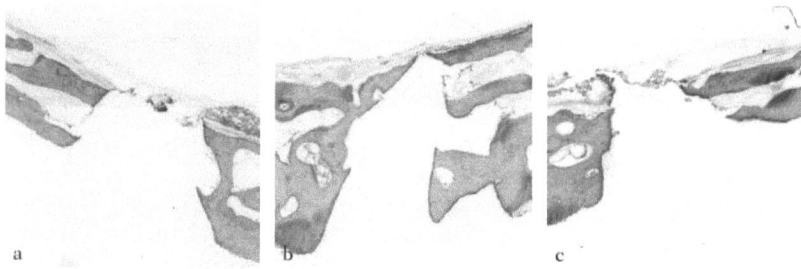

Figure 3.5: Transcrestal sinus osteotomy using laser devices may results in no (a), incomplete (b) or complete (c) maxillary sinus membrane perforation depending on energy settings used.

4. BIOMECHANICS OF TRANSCRESTAL SINUS MEMBRANE ELEVATION

4.1. Background

In transcrestal sinus floor elevation techniques, elevation forces must be high enough to facilitate membrane detachment without exceeding its deformation capacity. To predictably avoid membrane perforation it may prove worthwhile to pre-operatively assess the maximum elevation height that can safely be acchieved. The maximum height of transcrestal membrane elevation is correlated to [1] the three-dimensional internal anatomy of the maxillary sinus, [2] the elastic properties of the sinus membrane and quality of attachment to the underlying bony sinus floor (Berengo et al. 2004) and [3] the surgical technique used for transcrestal membrane elevation (Figure 4.1).

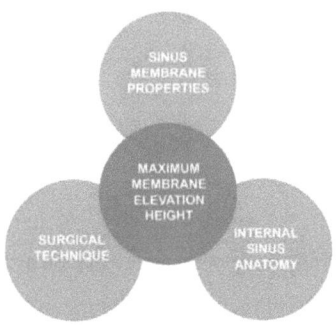

Figure 4.1: Factors related to the maximum height of transcrestal membrane elevation.

Three-dimensional internal anatomy of the maxillary sinus underlies significant interindividual variations. The size of the maxillary sinus has been found to vary between 3.5 and 35 cm³ (Ariji et al. 1994, Uchida et al. 1998) and the angle formed by the inner buccal and palatal alveolar walls of the sinus may range between 22° and 76° (Velloso et al. 2006). According to their mediolateral width, narrow sinuses (<30°), medium sinuses (31-60°) and wide sinuses (>60°) may be differentiated and show a frequency distribution of 17%, 29% and 54%, respectively (Cho et al. 2001). In cases of narrow internal sinus anatomy the circumference of the elevated subantral space is generally smaller compared to wider sinuses. As a consequence, the force required for membrane detachment is also relatively low and thus higher transcrestal membrane elevation may be acchieved in narrow sinuses (Figure 4.2).

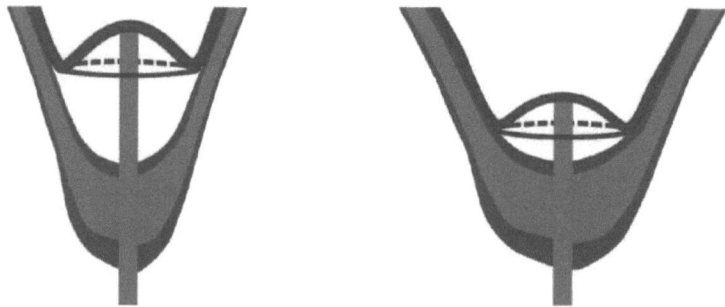

Figure 4.2: Narrow internal sinus anatomy (a) allows for higher transcrestal membrane elevation compared to wider sinuses (b) due to the smaller circumference of the elevated area.

Due to the elliptic profile of the maxillary sinus, the saggital angle between the anterior and posterior sinus wall is greater than the transverse angle between the buccal and palatal wall. Thus higher detachment forces must be expected in the saggital direction and the majority of membrane perforations can therefore be seen to extend from the buccal to the palatal sinus wall (Figure 4.3).

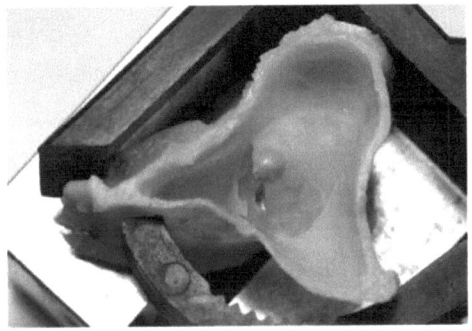

Figure 4.3: Sinus membrane perforation in transverse orientation.

Additional anatomic risk factors for membrane perforation comprise previous sinus surgery (ten Bruggenkate & van den Bergh 1998), absence of bone between the sinus membrane and the oral mucosa (Watzak et al. 2005), and irregularities of the bony sinus floor, such as the presence of maxillary sinus septa (Ulm et al. 1995).

Maxillary sinus septa are barriers of cortical bone that divide the maxillary sinus floor into multiple compartments, known as recesses. Today's knowledge on paranasal sinus anatomy is largely based on the work of Austrian anatomist Emil Zuckerkandl in the late 1800s (Stammberger

1989), however, maxillary sinus septa were first analyzed regarding their prevalence and characteristics by Arthur S. Underwood, an anatomist at King's College London, and are thus also referred to as Underwood's septa (Underwood 1910). They are thought to strengthen the sinus structure and act as masticatory force carrying struts (van den Bergh et al. 2000). Antral septa constitute partly congenital and partly acquired anatomic variations. They can be classified as either primary (developmental) or secondary septa, i.e. remnants from irregular sinus pneumatization (Krennmair et al. 1997) frequently leaving the sinus floor anterior and posterior to the septum at different levels. While septa located apical to a dentate alveolar ridge are primary, it is impossible to label septa located apical to edentulous ridges as either primary or secondary without previous radiographic records (Kim et al. 2006). Incomplete septa have been defined as at least 2.5 mm in height (Ulm et al. 1995) and are not thought to alter sinus drainage. In certain cases, however, septa may completely divide the sinus into two cavities (draining into the nose via separate openings (Selcuk et al. 2008).

While maxillary sinus septa have thus been considered clinically insignificant variations for decades, they have gained practical relevance for periodontists, oral and maxillofacial surgeons as well as otolaryngologists (Rysz & Bakoń 2009). Septa may hamper visibility in sinus endoscopy via a transnasal approach (Gosau et al. 2009) and interfere with surgical procedures like polypectomy and endoscopic removal of foreign bodies or tooth roots (Rosano et al. 2010). Sinus septa have become increasingly important after the introduction of sinus floor augmentation surgery (Boyne & James 1980) as they may complicate both creation and inversion of the access window in the lateral sinus wall, as well as elevation of the sinus membrane from the bony sinus floor (Betts & Miloro 1994). The presence of sinus septa is generally associated with a higher risk of membrane perforation (Shibli et al. 2007). Stronger adhesion of the sinus membrane to the knife edged septa has been postulated as a possible cause (Chanavaz 1990). Scarce data on results of sinus floor elevation in cases of sinus septa indicates a perforation rate of 26% on average (Kasabah et al. 2003, Toscano et al. 2010, Zijderveld et al. 2008), yet no study has demonstrated significant differences compared to sinuses without septa (χ^2 of combined data from the 3 studies = 1.178, p=0.278).

While maxillary sinus anatomy and the thickness of the maxillary sinus membrane represent fixed risk factors for membrane perforation, the risk of rupture may be reduced by modification of the surgical elevation techniques. As can be seen in Figure 4.4, the critical perforation force depends on the surgical technique used for transcrestal membrane elevation, i.e., on the area of force transmission. In osteotome-mediated membrane elevation (Summers 1994), the area of force transmission is equal to the surface area at the proximal end of the osteotome. Therefore, higher forces can safely be applied using osteotomes with large diameters for elevation due to the better load transfer.

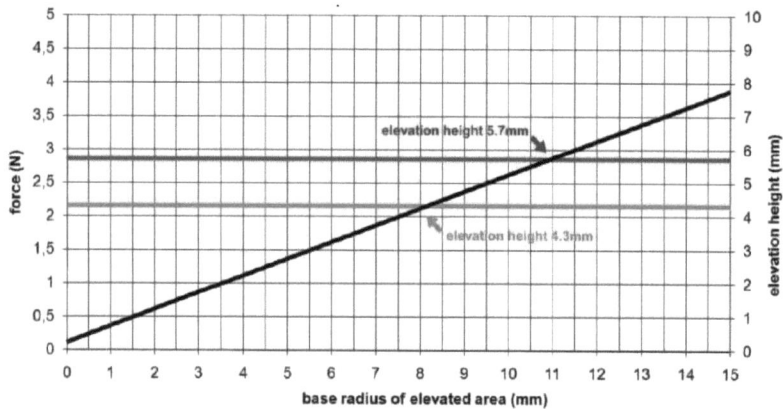

Figure 4.4: Required detachment force for sinus membrane elevation of 1-8 mm (black line); maximum membrane elevation height using osteotomes with a diameter of 3 mm (green line) vs. osteotomes with a diameter of 4 mm (red line).

The point of intersection between the solid black and the dashed line in Figure 4.4 indicates the maximum height of membrane elevation that can be obtained with 4-mm osteotomes, as the force required for detachment may exceed the critical membrane perforation force if further membrane elevation was attempted. In the case of membrane elevation by balloon catheter inflation (Soltan & Smiler 2005) a larger area of force transmission may be achieved. But the inflated balloon may not always be in full contact with the sinus membrane during the elevation procedure (Figure 4.5b). Membrane elevation by hydraulic pressure (Chen & Cha 2005) or gel pressure (Pommer & Watzek 2009) has the inherent advantage of maximum force transmission area during the entire elevation procedure (Figure 4.5c). Compared with osteotome-mediated techniques (Figure

4.5a), in which the elevation forces are transferred to the sinus membrane by point transmission at any stage of the procedure, the area of force transmission increases in the course of fluid pressure-mediated elevation. Point forces that might cause membrane perforation are thus avoided. Experimental ex-vivo results indicate that 82% of the perforations during osteotome-mediated elevation are caused by point forces at the tip of the osteotome (Stelzle et al. 2009). The main advantage of the fluid pressure-mediated techniques is the smooth transfer of elevation forces. Compared with hydraulic elevation techniques using water as a medium of force transfer, sudden pressure that may cause membrane perforation is absorbed by the cushioning effect of the highly viscous hydroxypropyl methylcellulose. This is of particular importance at the end of the elevation procedure when the force required for detachment approaches the critical perforation force.

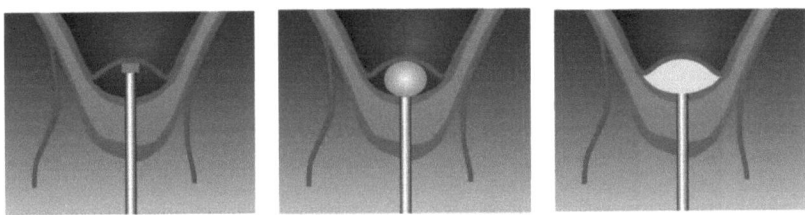

Figure 4.5: Transcrestal sinus membrane elevation by the use of osteotomes (a) , balloon inflation (b) or liquid pressure (c).

4.2. Biomechanical Properties of the Maxillary Sinus Membrane – Material and Methods

The aim of the following study was to investigate the mechanical properties of the maxillary sinus membrane in human cadaver specimen (Pommer et al. 2009). Detailed knowledge on the load limits of the membrane may help avoiding iatrogenic perforations during transcrestal maxillary sinus floor elevation and thus lowering the complication rate of the procedure.

The sample material comprised 20 unfixed human cadavers (10 male and 10 female subjects, age ranging from 56 to 87 years) that had been obtained from the Anatomical Institute of Vienna Medical University, Austria. By careful dissection the membrane samples were derived from the facial wall and floor of both maxillary sinuses immediately before experimentation. Time between testing and sample retrieval was kept to a minimum in order to preserve the elastic properties of the samples. The tissues were kept moistened in physiologic saline at room temperature to prevent dehydration. Three different types of sample specimen were obtained, 10 x 20 mm membrane stripes (n=39), 20 x 20 mm membrane squares (n=39) and 10 x 20 mm bone stripes with the sinus membrane still attached (n=22), for the three test methods planned. Two independent investigators assessed the thickness of the membrane stripes and squares in the center of the membrane samples using an electronic micrometer caliper accurate to 1 mm (Micromasters, Capa System, Switzerland).

The mechanical properties of the Schneiderian membrane, i.e . sinus membrane thickness, one- and two-dimensional burst elongation, one-and two-dimensional burst tension, modulus of elasticity and force of adhesion to the bone, were investigated by three test methods using a tensile tester.

[1] One-dimensional elongation (Figure 4.6): a total of 39 membrane stripes of 10 x 20 mm were clamped on both ends in an undilated position and stretched stepwise in increments of 1 mm until membrane perforation.

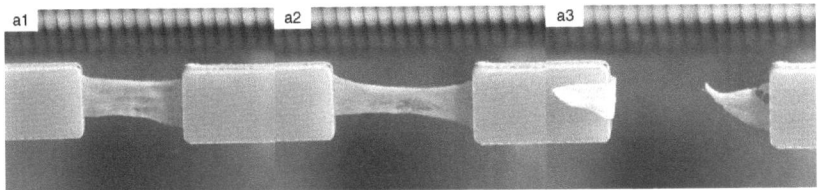

Figure 4.6: One-dimensional membrane elongation test.

[2] Two-dimensional elongation (Figure 4.7): a total of 39 membrane squares of 20 x 20 mm were mounted between clamping rings and centrally stretched by a spherical plunger of 3mm diameter until perforation.

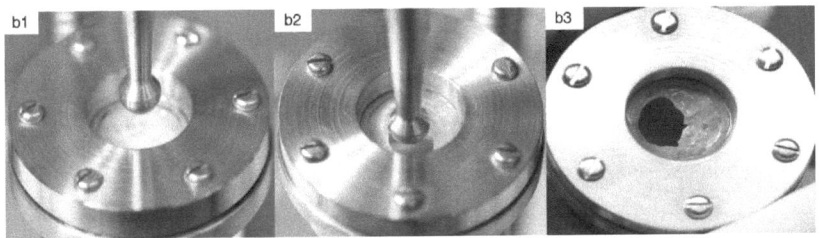

Figure 4.7: Two-dimensional membrane elongation test.

[3] Membrane detachment (Figure 4.8): sinus wall bone stripes of 10 x 20mm were installed into a mounting medium with the adherent membrane

gripped in a clamp on one end and elevated continuously until complete detachment.

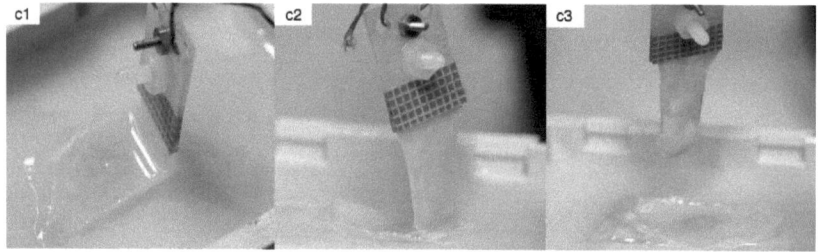

Figure 4.8: Membrane detachment test.

A load cell between moving and fixed probe holder recorded the tensile force. Counting the increments of the stepper motor with a constant speed of 1 mm/s (Roodenburg et al. 1990) the change in length was measured. Following membrane characteristics were computed based on the load-elongation curves recorded during the elongation tests: burst elongation (increase in length from start of the test until membrane perforation), burst tension (maximum load at the event of membrane perforation), and modulus of elasticity (amount of tension per extent of elongation). The adhesion force between the underlying bone and the Schneiderian membrane was calculated from the load measured in the course of the membrane detachment test.

For each test method mean values and standard deviations were calculated. A mixed effect model with fixed factors 'membrane thickness' and 'test method' and random factor 'specimen' was used for comparison of one- versus two-dimensional elongation. Variance estimation was performed separately for each test due to differing variances in the two tests. P-values were considered significant if found to be smaller than 0.05. All calculations were performed using R-project software (R Foundation for Statistical Computing, Vienna, Austria).

4.3. Biomechanical Properties of the Maxillary Sinus Membrane – Study Results

The membrane samples showed a mean thickness of 90 ± 45 µm (ranging from 24 µm to 350 µm). The inter-observer variability did not exceed 5 µm. No difference between the one- and two- dimensional test group regarding membrane thickkess could be found. Mean values of burst elongation in one-dimensional testing measured 32.6 ± 12.3% (ranging between 16.7% and 74.7%) and 24.7 ± 4.7% (ranging from 15.2% to 35.5%) in two-dimensional testing. Mean values of burst elongation were significantly lower in two-dimensional testing compared to one-dimensional testing (p=0.002). Thickness of the membrane samples showed a highly significant influence on burst elongation (p<0.001). Burst tension at the event of membrane perforation measured on average 7.3 ± 4.2 N/mm² (ranging between 2.3 N/mm² and 12.5 N/mm²). No statistically significant difference between the two test methods could be observed regarding burst tension. The Schneiderian membrane's modulus of elasticity was 0.058 ± 0.03 GPa on average (ranging from 0.012 GPa to 0.185 GPa). Differences between the elastic modulus in one- and two-dimensional elongation could not be found to be statistically significant. The force of adhesion between the maxillary sinus membrane and the bony maxillary sinus floor ranged between 0.015 N/mm and 0.103N/mm with a mean of 0.05 ± 0.025N/mm. Descriptive statistics of all measurments can be found in Table 4.1:

	one-dimensional elongation (n=39)	two-dimensional elongation (n=39)	membrane detachment (n=22)
membrane thickeness (mm)	0.099 ± 0.056	0.080 ± 0.028	–
burst elongation (%)	32.6 ± 12.3	24.7 ± 4.7	–
burst tension (N/mm^2)	5.9 ± 2.5	8.6 ± 5.1	–
modulus of elasticity (GPa)	0.049 ± 0.019	0.070 ± 0.04	–
adhesion force (N/mm)	–	–	0.050 ± 0.025

Table 4.1: Mechanical properties of the Schneiderian membrane: membrane thickeness, burst elongation, burst tension, modulus of elasticity and adhesion force (mean value ± standard deviation).

4.4. Impact of Surgical Technique and Internal Sinus Anatomy – Material and Methods

The aim of the following study (Pommer et al. 2013a) was to investigate the impact of the surgical technique used (osteotome-mediated vs. liquid/gel pressure-mediated membrane elevation) as well as the impact of the internal sinus anatomy on maximum height of transcrestal membrane elevation. Analyses were based on three-dimensional computed tomographic data and on the biomechanical properties of the maxillary sinus membrane (cf. chapters 4.2 and 4.3) that had been assessed in the previous study (Pommer et al. 2009).

A total of nine computed tomographies of edentulous maxillae were selected according to their internal sinus anatomy, i.e. the angle between the buccal and the palatal sinus wall: 3 sinuses demonstrated narrow angles (less than 80°), 3 sinuses had angles between 80° and 100° and 3 sinuses demonstrated wide angles (larger than 100°). CT data was transferred to MiniMagics analytic software (V12.0.6.2, Materialise) to construct a three-dimensional surface model of the maxillary sinus using complex surface rendering (Figure 4.9). The site of transcrestal osteotomy was set at the lowest point of the maxillary sinus and distances to the four sinus walls (anterior, posterior, buccal, palatal) were measured on consecutive axial CT scans (slice thickness: 1 mm).

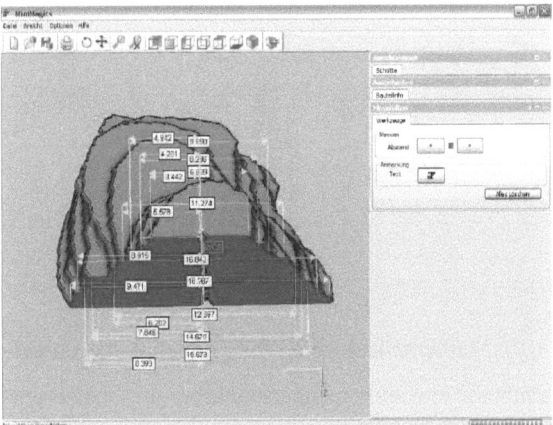

Figure 4.9: 3D complex surface rendering in MiniMagics analytic software.

Transcrestal sinus floor elevation was simulated based on a mathematical model. The maximum height of membrane elevation using osteotomes was calculated as follows: [1] $l_0=2*l_0'+D_O$; [2] $l_0'=(l_0-D_O)/2$; [3] $e_0=l_0'*1.247$; [4] $e_0^2=(l_0')^2+h_0^2$; [5] $h_0=\sqrt{e_0^2-(l_0')^2}$; [6] $l_1'=l_0'+z_1$; [7] $z_1^2=x_1^2+y_1^2$; [8] $x_1=(l_1-l_0)/2$; [9] $z_1=\sqrt{(l_1-l_0)^2+1^2}$; [10] $e_1=l_1'*1.247$; [11] $s_1=l_0+x_1$; [12] $e_1^2=s_1^2+(h_1')^2$; [13] $h_1'=\sqrt{e_1^2-s_1^2}$; [14] $h_1=h_1'+y_1$ and [15] $h_{ges}=h_x'+y_1+y_2+...y_x$, with D_O representing the diameter of the osteotome (in this analysis set to 3 mm), l_0 being the original length of the sinus membrane measured as the distance of the osteotome to the sinus wall and e_0 representing the length of the stretched sinus membrane assuming that it can safely be stretched to 124.7% of its original size without causing membrane perforation (Pommer et al. 2009). Calculation of the maximum elevation height using osteotomes were based on the Pythagorean theorem (Figure 4.10).

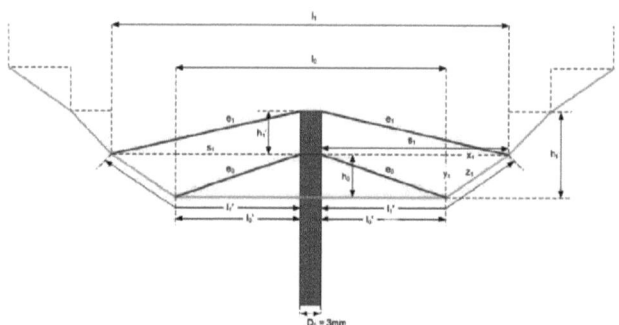

Figure 4.10: Mathematical model for simulation of transcrestal sinus membrane elevation using osteotomes of 3 mm diameter.

The maximum height of membrane elevation using liquid/gel pressure was calculated as follows: [1] $b_0=l_0*1.247$; [2] $l=2r*\sin(b/2r)$; [3] $l_0=2r_0*\sin(b_0/2r_0)$; [4] $r=l/2*\sin(b/2r)$; [5] $r_0=l_0/2*\sin(b_0/2r_0)$; [6] $r_0=f(r_0)$; [7] $b=r*a$; [8] $b_0=r_0*a_0$; [9] $a_0=b_0/r_0*180/p$; [10] $r_0^2=\Delta r_0^2+(l_0/2)^2$; [11] $h_0=r_0-\Delta r_0$; [12] $z_1^2=x_1^2+y_1^2$; [13] $x_1=(l_1-l_0)/2$; [14] $z_1=\sqrt{[(l_1-l_0)/2]^2+1^2}$; [15] $l_1'=l_0+2*z_1$; [16] $b_1=[l_0+2*z_1]*1.247$; [17] $r_1=l_1/2*\sin(b_1/2r_1)$; [18] $a_1=b_1/r_1*180/\pi$; [19] $r_1^2=\Delta r_1^2+(l_1/2)^2$; [20] $h_1=(r_1-\Delta r_1)+y_1$; and maximum elevation height again being $h_{ges}=h_x'+y_1+y_2+...y_x$ (Figure 4.11).

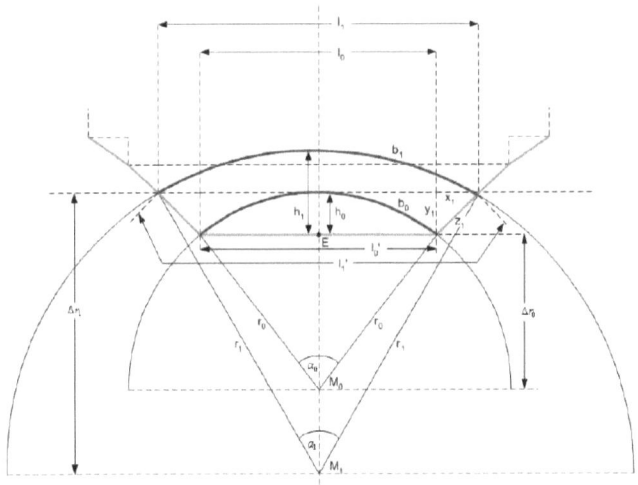

Figure 4.11: Mathematical model for simulation of transcrestal sinus membrane elevation using liquid/gel pressure.

According to the results of the previous study (cf. chapter 4.3) the biomechanical properties of the sinus membrane were set to: membrane thickness 90 μm, mebrane perforation occuring at a burst tension of 7.3

N/mm² and membrane adhesion force to the bony sinus floor being 0.05 N/mm (Pommer et al. 2009).

4.5. Impact of Surgical Technique and Internal Sinus Anatomy – Study Results

Mean height of maxillary sinus membrane elevation using osteotomes was lower compared to liquid- or gel-pressure (4.6 mm vs. 5.4 mm) in all investigated sinuses (Table 4.2). Differences ranged from 0.1 mm to 1.9 mm (mean: 0.8 mm). Narrow sinuses allowed for higher membrane elevation (5.8 ± 1.0 mm) than normal (5.5 ± 0.8 mm) or wide sinuses (5.0 ± 0.5 mm).

	internal angle	maximum height osteotomes	maximum height gel pressure	difference
narrow sinus anatomy	52°	4.2 mm	5.0 mm	0.8 mm
	66°	4.8 mm	5.2 mm	0.4 mm
	68°	5.3 mm	7.2 mm	1.9 mm
regular sinus anatomy	86°	6.3 mm	6.6 mm	0.3 mm
	89°	4.2 mm	4.8 mm	0.6 mm
	95°	4.1 mm	5.0 mm	0.9 mm
wide sinus anatomy	102°	4.3 mm	5.7 mm	1.4 mm
	112°	4.3 mm	4.4 mm	0.1 mm
	118°	4.1 mm	5.0 mm	0.9 mm
total	88 ± 21°	4.6 ± 0.7 mm	5.4 ± 0.9 mm	0.8 ± 0.5 mm

Table 4.2: Results of computed tomographic-based simulation of maximum height of sinus membrane elevation using osteotomes vs. gel-pressure in 9 cases of narrow (<80°), normal (80° to 100°) or wide (>100°) internal sinus anatomy.

Finite elemente analysis (FEA) allows for three-dimensional visualization of the simulated sinus membrane elevation procedures. While point forces causing membrane perforation can be seen at the tip of the osteotome (Figure 4.12) in osteotome-mediated elevation, even distribution of elevation forces can be seen in fluid or gel-pressure mediated procedures (Figure 4.13).

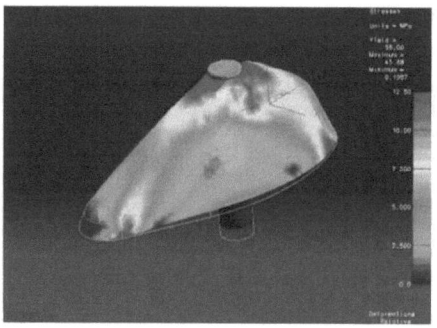

Figure 4.12: Finite elemente analysis (FEA) of transcrestal sinus membrane elevation using osteotomes. Point forces (red color) can be seen to occur around the tip of the osteotome.

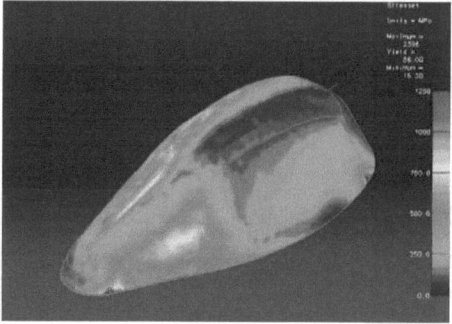

Figure 4.13: Finite elemente analysis (FEA) of transcrestal sinus membrane elevation using liquid- or gel-pressure. Even distribution of elevation forces can be appreciated.

4.6. Meta-Analysis of Maxillary Sinus Septa – Material and Methods

Prevalence of maxillary sinus septa in the literature ranges between 10% and 58% (Maestre-Ferrín et al. 2011, Yang et al. 2009). Recent literature reviews on the topic identified conflicting study results regarding not only overall prevalence, but also septa height, predominant septa location as well as prevalence in edentulism (Katranji et al. 2008, Maestre-Ferrín et al. 2010). Therefore, the aim of the following study was to gain further insights into prevalence, location and morphology of maxillary sinus septa using a meta-analytic approach (Pommer et al. 2012b).

A MEDLINE search of English literature (last search performed on June 1st 2011, key words: maxillary sinus septa, antral septa) was supplemented by hand searching the reference lists of all retrieved papers and relevant review articles (Katranji et al. 2008, Maestre-Ferrín et al. 2010, Rossetti et al. 2010). Studies were considered if they met the following inclusion criteria: [1] trials investigating maxillary sinus septa by 3D radiographic imaging or visual inspection in adults and [2] presenting data on septa prevalence per sinus. After exclusion of duplicates, 55 abstracts were screened. Full texts of 37 papers considered eligible for inclusion were obtained for further assessment against the stated criteria. Four publications were not written in English language (Lugmayr et al. 1996, Oh & Rue 1998, Qin & Li 1999, Xu et al. 2011), three studies did not meet inclusion criterion 1 (Maestre-Ferrín et al. 2010, Naitoh et al. 2010, Shibli et al. 2007), and five did not meet criterion 2 (Betts & Miloro 1994, Borris & Weber 1998, Fortin et al. 2011, Kfir et al. 2009, Meyers & Valvassori 1998).

Twenty-five trials constituted the final selection (Table 4.3) and underwent data abstraction. Authors of six studies were contacted for clarification or missing data. A total of 7263 sinuses were investigated: 6474 on computed tomographic images, 426 in human cadavers and 363 in patients undergoing sinus surgery. Prevalence data on gender differences were found in only five studies (Kim et al. 2006, Lee et al. 2010, Park et al. 2011, Shen et al. 2012, van Zyl & van Heerden 2009), differences between right and left sides were evaluated in eleven trials (Gosau et al. 2009, Kim et al. 2006, Koymen et al. 2009, Lee et al. 2010, Maestre-Ferrín et al. 2011, Neugebauer et al. 2010, Park et al. 2011, Selcuk et al. 2008, Shen et al. 2012, van Zyl & van Heerden 2009, Velásquez-Plata et al. 2002). Data on multiple septa per sinus was missing in seven investigations (Ella et al. 2008, Güncü et al. 2011, Kasabah et al. 2003, Park et al. 2011, Shen et al. 2012, Toscano et al. 2010, Zijderveld et al. 2008). Data on septa location was extracted from 14 studies (Table 4.4). In twelve publications it could not be clarified whether septa were located apical to dentate or edentulous ridges (Ella et al. 2008, Gosau et al. 2009, Güncü et al. 2011, Kasabah et al. 2002, Kasabah et al. 2003, Neugebauer et al. 2010, Park et al. 2011, Rysz & Bakoń 2009, Selcuk et al. 2008, Toscano et al. 2010, Yang et al. 2009, Zijderveld et al. 2008). Septa height was reported separately for dentate and edentulous subjects in four studies (Kim et al. 2006, Koymen et al. 2009, Maestre-Ferrín et al. 2011, Velásquez-Plata et al. 2002). Eleven papers did not provide the percentage of complete septa (Ella et al. 2008, Gosau et al. 2009, Güncü et al. 2011, Kasabah et al. 2002, Kasabah et al. 2003, Krennmair et al. 1999, Park et al. 2011, Rysz & Bakoń 2009, Selcuk et al. 2008, Toscano et al. 2010, Ulm et al. 1995) and ten studies did not investigate septa orientation (Ella et al. 2008, González-Santana et al. 2007, Gosau et al. 2009, Güncü et al. 2011, Kasabah et al. 2003, Krennmair et al. 1999, Lee et al. 2010, Rysz & Bakoń 2009, Toscano et al. 2010, Yang et al.

2009). Accuracy of panoramic radiographs in detecting sinus septa was evaluated in four trials (González-Santana et al. 2007, Kasabah et al. 2002, Krennmair et al. 1999, Maestre-Ferrín et al. 2011).

Septa prevalence is given as overall percentages with 95% confidence intervals. Weighted means of septa height and 95% confidence intervals were computed. Comparison of subgroups was performed using chi-square and independent two-sample t-tests, for prevalence and height data, respectively. Sensitivity (A/(A+C)) and specificity (D/(B+D)) of panoramic radiographs (PR) using computed tomography (CT) as a reference standard were calculated using absolute frequencies (A: septa visible in both CT and PR, B: septa visible in PR but not in CT, C: septa visible in CT but not in PR, D: septa not visible in both CT and PR). All analyses were performed using R 2.4.0 (R Foundation for Statistical Computing, Vienna, Austria).

4.7. Meta-Analysis of Maxillary Sinus Septa – Study Results

Septa were present in 28.8% [$CI^{95\%}$ 24.3-33.4] of 7263 maxillary sinuses investigated in 25 studies (Table 4.3). One quarter of patients (24.6% [$CI^{95\%}$ 18.0-31.1]) showed septa in one sinus (unilaterally), while 16.7% [$CI^{95\%}$ 11.5-21.9] featured septa bilaterally in both sinuses (n=3226). Two septa within the same sinus were observed in 3.7% [$CI^{95\%}$ 2.2-5.2], while only 0.5% [$CI^{95\%}$ 0.4-0.6] of sinuses had three or more septa (n=5323). Equal numbers of septa were reported in right (50.7%) and left (49.3%) sinuses (n=1986). Septa prevalence was significantly lower (p<0.001) in the Asian population (22.3%, n=1786) compared to Caucasian subjects (29.0%, n=5077), while no gender difference could be observed (p=0.207, n=1103).

While the majority of septa (54.6% [$CI^{95\%}$ 47.1-62.2]) were found in first or second maxillary molar regions, 24.4% [$CI^{95\%}$ 14.8-33.9] and 21.0% [$CI^{95\%}$ 14.8-27.2] were located in anterior (premolar) and posterior (retromolar) sinus regions, respectively (Table 4.4). Septa prevalence was significantly higher in edentulous ridges compared to dentate ridges (p<0.001, n=1167). Significant differences in septa distribution to anterior, middle and posterior regions were observed between dentate (27.1%, 58.6%, 14.3%) vs. edentulous ridges (12.6%, 69.5%, 17.9%) indicating increased prevalence in the region of the first and second molars following sinus pneumatization (p=0.007, n=339). Mean septa height measured 7.5 mm [$CI^{95\%}$ 6.7-8.4] (n=1686). No difference between septa height in dentate vs. edentulous ridges could be seen (p=0.902, n=339).

study	number of sinuses	sinuses with septa	unilateral septa	bilateral septa
Ella et al. 2008	150	33.3%	10.7%	28.0%
González-Santana et al. 2007	60	25.0%	23.3%	13.3%
Gosau et al. 2009	130	25.4%	23.1%	13.8%
Güncü et al. 2011	242	16.1%	n.d.	n.d.
Kasabah et al. 2002	68	35.3%	70.6%	0.0%
Kasabah et al. 2003	146	13.0%	n.d.	n.d.
Kim et al. 2006	200	26.5%	23.0%	15.0%
Koymen et al. 2009	410	35.4%	35.6%	17.6%
Krennmair et al. 1997	200	16.0%	10.0%	11.0%
Krennmair et al. 1999	102	29.4%	n.d.	n.d.
Lee et al. 2010	236	24.6%	25.5%	1.5%
Maestre-Ferrín et al. 2011	60	58.3%	43.3%	36.7%
Naitoh et al. 2009	30	36.7%	20.0%	26.7%
Neugebauer et al. 2010	2058	33.2%	27.7%	19.3%

Park et al. 2011	400	24.3%	25.5%	11.5%
Rosano et al. 2010	60	33.3%	13.3%	26.7%
Rysz & Bakoń 2009	222	22.1%	n.d.	n.d.
Selcuk et al. 2008	660	22.9%	19.1%	13.3%
Shen et al. 2012	846	20.4%	17.7%	11.6%
Toscano et al. 2010	56	30.4%	n.d.	n.d.
Ulm et al. 1995	41	31.7%	n.d.	n.d.
van Zyl & van Heerden 2009	400	55.5%	27.0%	42.0%
Velásquez-Plata et al. 2002	312	22.1%	21.2%	11.5%
Yang et al. 2009	74	9.5%	n.d.	n.d.
Zijderveld et al. 2008	100	48.0%	n.d.	n.d.
Total	7061	29.1%	24.6%	16.7%

Table 4.3: Prevalence of maxillary sinus septa per sinus in the 25 included studies as well as patient-based frequencies of uni- and bilateral sinus septa in 17 studies (n.d. = no data) as well as overall prevalence.

study	number of septa	anterior region	middle region	posterior region
Gosau et al. 2009	35	42.9%	51.4%	5.7%
Kim et al. 2006	59	25.4%	50.8%	23.7%
Koymen et al. 2009	165	18.8%	64.8%	16.4%
Krennmair et al. 1999	32	71.9%	28.1%	0.0%
Lee et al. 2010	66	27.3%	50.0%	22.7%
Maestre-Ferrín et al. 2011	40	17.5%	60.0%	22.5%
Neugebauer et al. 2010	814	23.1%	59.2%	17.7%
Park et al. 2011	111	22.5%	45.9%	31.5%
Rosano et al. 2010	20	30.0%	40.0%	30.0%
Shen et al. 2012	194	17.5%	54.1%	28.4%
Ulm et al. 1995	15	73.3%	26.7%	0.0%
van Zyl & van Heerden 2009	276	26.4%	48.9%	24.6%
Velásquez-Plata et al. 2002	75	24.0%	41.3%	34.7%
Yang et al. 2009	7	14.3%	85.7%	0.0%
Total	1909	24.4%	54.6%	21.0%

Table 4.4: Distribution of septa to anterior (premolar), middle (molar) and posterior (retromolar) sinus regions in 14 studies as well as overall distribution.

The vast majority of sinus septa (99.7% [$CI^{95\%}$ 99.1-100]) were incomplete, while only 0.3% [$CI^{95\%}$ 0.0-0.9] completely divided the sinus into 2 separate cavities (n=1825). Orientation of septa was transverse (buccopalatal) in 87.5% [$CI^{95\%}$ 78.4-96.7], saggital (mesiodistal) in 11.1% [$CI^{95\%}$ 2.1-20.2], and horizontal (parallel to the sinus floor) in 1.3% [$CI^{95\%}$

0.0-3.6] (n=2038). Transverse septa demonstrated significantly greater height at their medial (palatal) insertion compared to their lateral (buccal) aspect (6.9 mm vs. 4.1 mm, p=0.047, n=299). Diagnosis of sinus septa using panoramic radiographs yielded incorrect results in 29.3% [$CI^{95\%}$ 11.9-46.7] (n=249). Using CT scans as the reference standard, panoramic radiographs show a test sensitivity (true positive rate) of 53.8% [$CI^{95\%}$ 37.3-70.4] and a test specificity (true negative rate) of 80.4% [$CI^{95\%}$ 64.5-96.3].

4.8. Discussion

In transcrestal sinus augmentation techniques it is a great concern to avoid iatrogenic perforation of the maxillary sinus membrane, as membrane elevation is not performed under optic or tactile control and the access for membrane repair is limited (Toffler 2004). Membrane perforation in the course of maxillary sinus floor elevation can be attributed to inadequate surgical technique or to the presence of a thin sinus mucosa (Berengo et al. 2004). In the present human cadaver study (Pommer et al. 2009) membrane thickness ranged between 24 and 350 micrometer, so it can be concluded that the tested membranes were not pathologically thickened, and the biomechanical properties of the unfixed human cadaver membranes should be comparable to those in healthy organisms. Chronic maxillary sinusitis and allergic conditions can lead to a thickened mucosa (van den Bergh et al. 2000) and even in healthy patients variations in the thickness of the Schneiderian membrane of up to 800 mm have been observed (Morgensen & Tos 1977). Additional risk factors comprise previous sinus surgery (ten Bruggenkate & van den Bergh 1998), absence of bone between sinus mucosa and oral mucosa (Watzak et al. 2005), and irregularities of the bony sinus floor, such as maxillary sinus septa (Krennmair et al. 1997, Ardekian et al. 2006).

The overall prevalence of maxillary sinus septa (28.8% [$CI^{95\%}$ 24.3-33.4]) proved to be only slightly lower than the frequency of 33.3% reported one century ago (Underwood 1910). The present meta-analysis (Pommer et al. 2012b), however, gained further insights into rare characteristics, such as complete septa (0.3%), saggital (11.1%) or horizontal (1.3%) septa orientation, multiple septa per sinus (4.2%) and bilateral septa in both sinuses (16.7%). Potential limitations may arise from divergent criteria of septa definition throughout the included studies: 13 trials did not set a minimum septa size, while 12 investigations regarded only septa higher than 2-4 mm to exclude irregularities and uneven patches of the sinus floor from the analysis (Ulm et al. 1995). However, no significant difference in septa prevalence could be found between studies with vs. without restriction as well as between threshold definitions of <2.5 mm vs. ≥ 2.5 mm (p>0.05). Evaluation using 3D radiographic imaging vs. direct clinical observation yielded no significant different results (p=0.158). As radiographic investigations are frequently carried out in selected patient groups like those referred for implant treatment, recruitment bias may be assumed (Selcuk et al. 2008). This seems inevitable as radiation exposure calls for medico-ethical justification.

Compared to 3D computed tomography, diagnosis of sinus septa using 2D panoramic radiographs yield incorrect results in 29% of cases. Sinus septa showing a saggital orientation (Figure 4.14) may not be diagnosable at all using panoramic radiographs and may thus lead to assumption of narrow internal sinus anatomy and subsequent non-augmentation of the medial portion of the sinus cavity. The necessity of preoperative radiographic imaging should be judged on its therapeutic consequences, in case of sinus floor augmentation ranging from modification of the surgical access strategy or window design to change in implant positions or total avoidance of bone graft surgery. In view of the high overall prevalence and significant morphologic variability of sinus septa seen in the present investigation, 3D radiography prior to sinus floor augmentation surgery seems advisable on a regular basis.

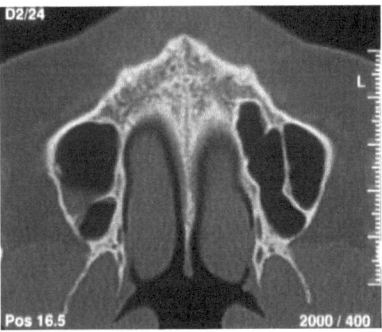

Figure 4.14: Axial CT scan of a patient with bilateral maxillary sinus septa showing transverse (buccopalatal) orientation on the right side and saggital (mesiodistal) orientation on the left side.

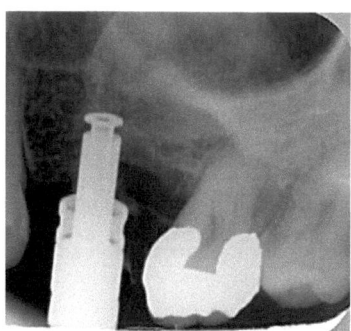

Figure 4.15: Intraoperative x-ray during transcrestal sinus floor elevation using the gel-pressure technique (Pommer & Watzek 2009) reveals distal deviation of membrane elevation due to the presence of a transverse sinus septum.

Transcrestal sinus floor elevation may be significantly complicated by maxillary sinus septa of any orientation (Gosau et al. 2009). Patterns of membrane elevation might be unpredictable in the presence of septa (Figure 4.15) and possibilities to diagnose or even repair sinus membrane perforations are limited (Pommer et al. 2009).

The present computed tomography-based analysis (Pommer et al. 2013a) revealed that maximum elevation heights are lower for osteotome- vs. liquid or gel pressure-mediated (4.6 mm vs. 5.4 mm on average). In literature, the average height of sinus elevation has been reported to range between 2.5 mm and 8.6 mm for transcrestal techniques (Nkenke et al. 2002, Engelke et al. 2003, Toffler 2004, Vitkov et al. 2005, Ferrigno et al. 2006, Nedir et al. 2006). In the course of transcrestal sinus floor elevation, the force needed for further sinus membrane detachment increases with the size of the already elevated area. In other words, the force required for detachment to gain an elevation of 3 mm is relatively low, while advancing membrane elevation from 3 to 6 mm necessitates higher force levels. The detachment force (at any time of the elevation procedure) may be calculated by multiplying the force of adhesion between the sinus membrane and the underlying bone (0.05 N/mm) by the circumference of the elevated area. As soon as the force required for detachment exceeds the stress tolerance limit of the sinus membrane, perforation may occur. The critical perforation force of the sinus membrane can be calculated by multiplying the membrane burst tension (7.3 N/mm^2) by the area of force transmission. As the detachment force is correlated to the circumference of the elevated area, and the three-dimensional sinus anatomy significantly varies interindividually, the maximum elevation height obtainable with transcrestal techniques differs from patient to patient.

Three-dimensional computed tomographic imaging provides quantitative information on the precise maxillary sinus anatomy (Gahleitner et al. 2003). Information on the individual internal sinus anatomy allows for preopeative assessment of the maximum height of transcrestal sinus membrane elevation specific to a certain patient case (Pommer & Watzek 2009). If membrane elevation is accomplished by baloon- or gel-pressure-techniques, it is possible to determine the amount of fluid that needs to be injected to acchieve the intended height of membrane elevation. By this means, the volume of bone graft material required may be ascertained prior to sinus augmentation. Due to the optimized force transmission, the height of membrane elevation achievable with the gel-pressure technique is superior to the amount of elevation obtainable with osteotomes.

In cases of two or more adjacent implants to be placed in combination with transcrestal sinus floor augmentation, membrane elevation may be performed via multiple access osteotomies. Separate subantral spaces are created apical to each osteotomy at the beginning of the elevation procedure. At some point – dependent on the mesiodistal space between the osteotomies – the adjacent subantral spaces may merge to one combined space. If the same amount of membrane elevation is carried out via two adjacent osteotomies at the same speed, the two corresponding subantral spaces merge half-way in between the osteotomies (Figure 4.16a), as membrane detachent occurs concentrically around each osteotomy. If elevation is performed predominantly via one of the osteotomies, the merging point is situated off-centered closer to the second osteotomy (Figure 4.16b).

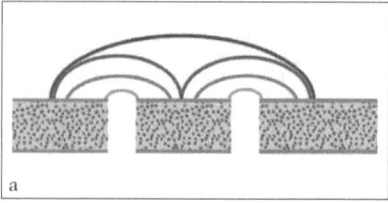 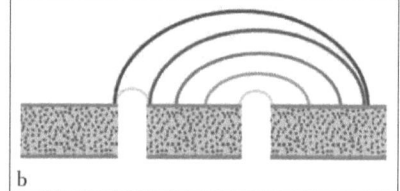

Figure 4.16: Fig. 8: (a) central merging point of two adjacent subantral spaces, (b) off-centered merging point of two adjacent subantral spaces.

Differences in timing and amount of elevation between the two adjacent osteotomies may thus result in different shapes of the combined subantral space (Figure 4.16). Furthermore it must be respected that the bony floor of the maxillary sinus is usually concave and characterized by an inclined anterior border in the premolar region in 55% of cases (Kim et al. 2003).

Advanced membrane elevation via the mesial osteotomy will therefore produce greater elevation heights and a mesial-shift of the resulting subantral space (Figure 4.17a). By contrast, a flatter and distally-shifted elevation pattern can be seen if the distal osteotomy is chosen as a starting point for membrane detachment (Figure 4.17b).

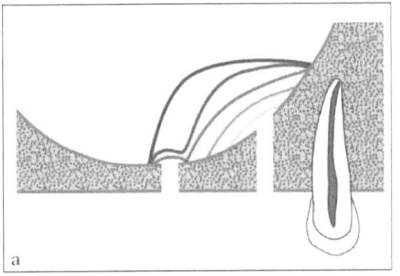 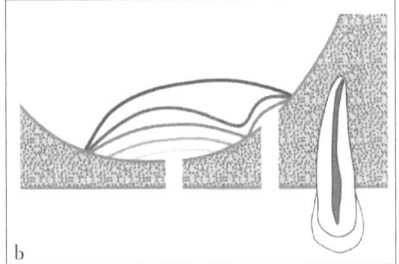

Figure 4.17: Patterns of membrane elevation in case of initial elevation via the mesial (a) or the distal (b) of two transcrestal access osteotomy.

If a total of three or more access osteotomies are carried out simultaneously, it may be preferable to start membrane elevation via the most mesial and most distal osteotomy (Figure 4.18). Compared to a cental starting point, this course of action may enable greater membrane elevation heights without risking membrane perforation, and thus placement of higher bone graft volumes.

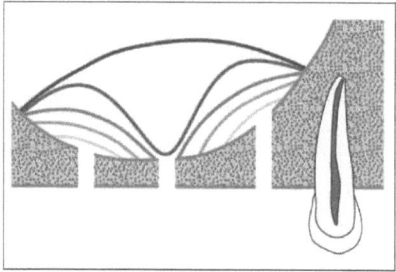

Figure 4.18: Membrane elevation pattern in case of 3 access osteotomies.

5. SIMULTANEOUS IMPLANT PLACEMENT AND PRIMARY IMPLANT STABILITY

5.1. Background

The surgical technique of transcrestal maxillary sinus floor augmentation as originally described by Summers (Summers 1994) involves simultaneous placement of dental implants into the transcrestal osteotomy. The inherent advantages of one-stage implant placement are not only a reduction of surgical interventions but also a reduction of postoperative healing periods, and thus total treatment time, by half. In techniques that do not use any kind of bone graft material and aim to initiate bone formation exclusively by maxillary sinus membrane elevation and blood clot formation underneath, implants play an essential role as they serve as tent poles for the sinus membrane. In flapless transcrestal elevation techniques (Pommer & Watzek 2009) implants are routinely placed simultaneously and subjected to transmucosal healing.

It is consequently of uttermost importance that simultaneously placed implants reach sufficient primary stability despite the fact that they will only have contact to the residual alveolar bone at their coronal aspect and not at the full implant length as usual. Low initial stability (smaller than 20 Ncm) carries an increased risk of osseointegration failure and transmucosal healing may even increase that risk due to implant micromotions during the healing period. While investigations using resonance frequency analysis found that the marginal ridge of the bony sinus floor is most important in the provision of stability, it is still not completely understood what minimum amount of residual bone height is actually needed to retain implants placed in conjunction with transcrestal sinus floor augmentation (Thor et al. 2007). In studying the effects of residual alveolar ridge height on primary implant stability it is important to also include local jawbone quality as a confounding factor in the analysis, as bone density may decrease along with progressive sinus pneumatization. In addition, it may be possible to compensate the reduced bone-to-implant contact surface – and thus enhance primary implant stability – by increasing the diameter of implants in the presence of compromised alveolar height in the posterior maxilla.

5.2. Primary Implant Stability – Material & Methods

The aim of the following study was to investigate the impact of residual alveolar ridge height, radiographic bone density and implant diameter on primary stability of implants placed in the sinus floor of atrophic human cadaver maxillae (Pommer et al. 2012c).

Edentulous maxillae of 11 fresh human cadavers (mean age: 79 years) were obtained from the Institute of Anatomy (Vienna Medical University, Austria). No formaldehyde fixation was carried out to avoid alteration in tissue consistency. All included subjects were free from bone pathology and stored at 4°C following radiographic examination (O'Sullivan et al. 2000). Computed tomographic scans were acquired with a conventional CT scanner (Tomoscan SR-6000, Philips, Eindhoven, the Netherlands) using a standard dental CT investigation protocol: 1.5mm slice thickness, 1.0 mm table feed, 120 kV, 75 mA, 2 s scan time, 100-120 mm field of view, high-resolution bone filter (Gahleitner et al. 2003). Residual alveolar ridge height was assessed at three designated implant sites (anterior, middle, posterior) per side and average radiographic bone density within each area was computed in Hounsfield Units (HU). Gutta-percha markers were used to determine the designated implant sites clinically at insertion (Figure 5.1, Figure 5.2). Measurements were performed using the Easy Vision Workstation (Philips, Eindhoven, the Netherlands).

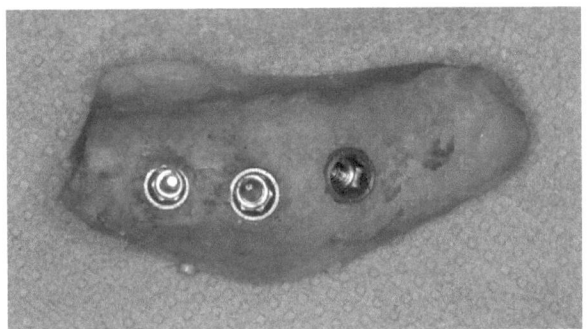

Figure 5.1: Implants placed in residual alveolar ridge of cadaver maxillae (coronal view).

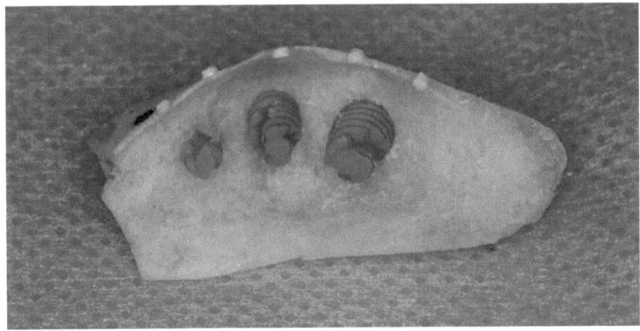

Figure 5.2: Implants placed in residual alveolar ridge of cadaver maxillae (apical view).

Following retraction of a mucoperiosteal flap a total of 66 NobelActive® implants (NA Internal, TiUnite, Nobel Biocare AB, Göteborg, Sweden) 10 mm in length were placed. Each of the 22 posterior maxillary segements received 3 implants: 1 narrow diameter implant (3.5 mm), 1 regular diameter implant (4.3 mm) and 1 wide diameter implant (5.0 mm). Implants were placed in the anterior, middle or posterior site according to their diameter to acchieve the most even distribution possible regarding residual alveolar ridge height grouped into 4 categories: 2.0-2.9 mm, 3.0-3.9 mm, 4.0-4.9 mm and 5.0-6.0 mm (Table 5.1).

residual alveolar ridge height	narrow diameter (3.5 mm)	regular diameter (4.3 mm)	wide diameter (5.0 mm)	total
2.0-2.9 mm	4 (6%)	4 (6%)	2 (3%)	10 (15%)
3.0-3.9 mm	6 (9%)	5 (8%)	7 (11%)	18 (27%)
4.0-4.9 mm	8 (12%)	7 (11%)	6 (9%)	21 (32%)
5.0-6.0 mm	4 (6%)	6 (9%)	7 (11%)	17 (26%)
total	22 (33%)	22 (33%)	22 (33%)	66 (100%)

Table 5.1: Absolute and relative (%) distribution of implant diameters regarding residual alveolar ridge height.

Primary implant stability was evaluated by [1] cutting resistance measurement during implant insertion using a INTRAsurg® 1000 surgical unit (KaVo, Bieberach, Germany) to record insertion torque values (ITVs) via wLink Control wireless data transfer (Figure 5.3), [2] damping capacity assessment using Periotest® (Siemens AG, Bensheim, Germany) that produces more negative Periotest values (PTVs) to indicate greater stability (Noguerol et al. 2006), and [3] resonance frequency analysis (RFA) using

Osstell® mentor (Integration Diagnostics AB, Gothenburg, Sweden) and Smartpeg™ type 21 and 47 abutments to measure implant stability quotient (ISQ) values (Karl et al. 2008).

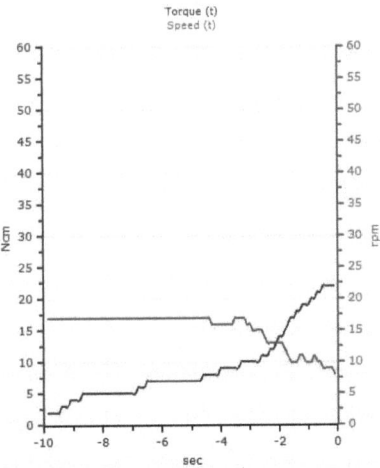

Figure 5.3: Increasing insertion torque values (Ncm, blue curve) and decreasing speed (rpm, green curve) recorded during implant placement.

Peak ITVs (Ncm) constituted the primary outcome variable, while PTVs and ISQs were secondary outcomes and assessed repeatedly, according to the manufacturers' recommendations. Differences in alveolar bone height distribution regarding implant diameters were investigated using chi-square testing. Linear relationship within the outcome variables was tested using Spearman's correlation coefficient and associated p-values considered to be significant if smaller than 0.05. Association of the 3 outcome variables to residual alveolar ridge height, radiographic bone density as well as implant diameter, respectively, were tested by multifactorial analysis of variance (ANOVA) at a Bonferoni-corrected significance level of 0.05/3=0.017. Statistical analyses were performed using R-project software (R Foundation for Statistical Computing, Vienna, Austria).

5.3. Primary Implant Stability – Study Results

Mean residual alveolar ridge height at the implant sites measured 4.0 ± 1.4 mm (range: 2-6 mm). Anterior, middle and posterior sinus segments offered mean bone heights of 4.0 ± 1.2 mm, 4.1 ± 1.5 mm and 4.1 ± 1.2 mm, respectively. Mean radiographic bone density measured 110 ± 51 HU (range: 34-239 HU). Ten implant sites (15%) showed residual bone heights between 2.0 and 2.9 mm (mean HU: 133 ± 42), 18 sites (27%) between 3.0 and 3.9 mm (mean HU: 112 ± 55), 21 sites (32%) between 4.0 and 4.9 mm (mean HU: 104 ± 45) and 17 sites (26%) between 5.0 and 6.0 mm (mean HU: 104 ± 63). No correlation between residual alveolar bone height and radiographic bone density could be observed ($r_s=0.21$, p=0.094).

Distribution of implant diameters regarding residual alveolar bone height was homogenous (Table 5.1) and demonstrated no significant differences ($\chi^2=2.24$, p=0.896). Narrow-, regular- and wide-diameter implants were placed in bone with a mean density of 125 ± 55 HU, 108 ± 52 HU and 99 ± 46 HU, respectively. Mean ITVs measured 17.0 ± 7.8 Ncm (range: 5-38 Ncm). PTVs ranged between -2 and 27 with an average of 8 ± 7. Mean ISQ values were 44 ± 12 (range: 8-70). Descriptive analysis of results regarding residual bone height and implant diameter is presented in Table 5.2. Correlations between the three outcome parameters (ITV vs. PTV: $r_s=-0.58$, ITV vs. ISQ: $r_s=0.52$, PTV vs. ISQ: $r_s=-0.73$) were all highly significant (p<0.001).

	residual alveolar bone height			
	2.0-2.9 mm	3.0-3.9 mm	4.0-4.9 mm	5.0-6.0 mm
insertion torque				
3.5 mm	19 ± 12	16 ± 8	16 ± 7	20 ± 9
4.3 mm	19 ± 5	14 ± 10	16 ± 6	14 ± 8
5.0 mm	16 ± 9	17 ± 6	19 ± 13	16 ± 7
Periotest® value				
3.5 mm	8 ± 6	8 ± 8	6 ± 6	2 ± 3
4.3 mm	7 ± 6	11 ± 12	12 ± 9	5 ± 4
5.0 mm	14 ± 16	7 ± 5	8 ± 7	9 ± 6
ISQ (Osstell®)				
3.5 mm	45 ± 19	45 ± 22	50 ± 11	61 ± 8
4.3 mm	34 ± 7	37 ± 12	42 ± 6	46 ± 5
5.0 mm	42 ± 4	45 ± 9	37 ± 16	46 ± 3

Table 5.2: Descriptive analysis of outcome measure values (insertion torque value, Periotest value, implant stability quotient (ISQ) of Osstell® measurements) regarding residual bone height groups and implant diameters (3.5 mm, 4.3 mm and 5.0 mm).

Among the three influencing variables, only radiographic bone density demonstrated statistically significant correlations to ITVs, PTVs as well as ISQ values at a Bonferoni-corrected level of $p<0.017$ in multifactorial ANOVA (Table 5.3). The highest degree of association was found between bone density and ITVs ($r_s=0.64$, $p<0.001$). The inverse correlation between bone density and PTVs ($r_s=-0.44$, $p>0.001$) goes to show that high bone density is associated with low PTVs, i.e. high implant stability. The correlation between ISQ values and bone density ($r_s=0.29$, $p=0.018$) was weak, however significant. No association to any of the three outcome measures could be found for both residual alveolar bone height as well as implant diameter.

	residual bone height	bone density	implant diameter
insertion torque	-0.03 (p=0.781)	0.64 (p<0.001) *	-0.01 (p=0.966)
Periotest® value	-0.11 (p=0.374)	-0.44 (p<0.001) *	0.19 (p=0.136)
ISQ (Osstell®)	0.29 (p=0.018)	0.39 (p=0.001) *	-0.25 (p=0.043)

Table 5.3: Results of multifactorial ANOVA (analysis of variance): correlation coefficients and p-values showing associations of influencing variable (bone density, residual bone height, implant diameter) and outcome measures (insertion torque value, Periotest value, implant stability quotient (ISQ) of Osstell® measurements) of primary implant stability (* indicating statistical significance at a Bonferoni-corrected level of p<0.017).

5.4. Discussion

Study results yielded local jawbone quality to be the major determinant of primary stability of implants placed in alveolar ridges of 2 to 6 mm height. Bone density (measured on preoperative computed tomographies) consistently demonstrated significant correlations to all three outcome measures that were used to assess primary implant stability, i.e. insertion torque values (ITV), Periotest® values (PTV) as well as implant stability quotient (ISQ) values. ITV measurements, however, revealed the highest degree of correlation. This finding is in line with the results of a recent study comparing primary stability measurements to bone quality parameters assessed in unfixed human cadaver jawbone using micro-CTs (Akça et al. 2006) that also found insertion torque values to be most sensitive in terms of revealing biomechanical properties at the bone-implant interface.

An experimental trial of similar design was performed in eight mini pigs to investigate bone-to-implant contacts 6 months after maxillary sinus floor augmentation via a lateral approach and simultaneous implant placement (Fenner et al. 2005). Residual alveolar bone height was reduced to 2 mm, 4 mm, 6 mm and 8 mm in 2 of the animals, respectively, prior to implant placement (Figure 5.4). Primary implant stability was not measured in this trial and comparisons were drawn between pigs rather than within the same animal. In the present study – comparing all three implant diameters within the same sinus – all possible attempts were made to guarantee an even distribution of implant diameters regarding not only residual alveolar bone height but also radiologic bone density. Statistical analyses did not indicate any signs of heterogenity, however, suboptimal homogeneity in the distribution of implants represents a practical limitation of the present study design. The only possibility to circumvent this issue would have been a reduction of alveolar bone to the desired height (as described by Fenner et al.), on the other hand, removal of bone cortex (either crestal cortical bone or the cortex of the bony sinus floor) would have altered bone structure significantly and carried the risk of introducing measurement bias.

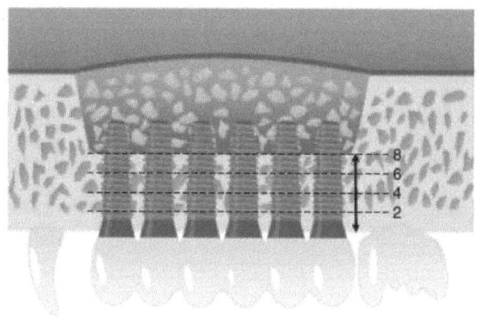

Figure 5.4: Reduction of the bony sinus floor to the desired residual alveolar bone height in an experimental animal trial (Fenner et al. 2005).

Primary stability is naturally related to the method of implant site preparation. In the present cadaver study predrilling of the implant bed was performed according to the recommendations of the manufacturer in the presence of low bone quality (type IV bone). These guidelines, however, have been established for the use in conventional cases and there are no separate manufacturer guidelines – nor any recommendations from the scientific community – regarding changes in implant bed preparation for simultaneous implants in reduced residual bone heights of 2-6 mm. Surgical options to adapt site preparation in cases of low bone quality in order to increase resulting primary stability involve (a) the underpreparation technique, i.e. not using drills to their full length or either not using final drills at all, or (b) the use of tapered osteotomes to laterally condense bone and create a denser interface at the placed implants (O'Sullivan et al. 2004). The suggestion of the present study that low primary stability may be predictable by preoperative radiographic bone density measurements provides implications for future research. Study results on the effectiveness of adapted implant site preparation to ensure satisfactory primary stability of simultaneous implants – as well as on the difference between different techniques (osteotome vs. underpreparation) – may help to establish guidelines that specify how to best react on the diagnosis of low bone quality in preoperative computed tomography.

6. BONE REGENERATION AND IMPACT ON SINUS PHYSIOLOGY

6.1. Background

While recent clinical and preclinical research has mainly focused on (histo)morphological aspects of bone regeneration following maxillary sinus floor augmentation surgery (Busenlechner et al. 2009), little is known on maxillary sinus compliance (Pignataro et al. 2008), i.e. the intrinsic potential of the maxillary sinus membrane to resume its homeostatic status following the iatrogenic surgical trauma caused by sinus membrane elevation and sinus floor augmentation. Termination of mucociliary activity was recently revealed by intraoperative nasal endoscopy in detached areas of the maxillary sinus membrane once elevated from the bony sinus floor (Griffa et al. 2010). While absence of inflammatory membrane response following bone graft consolidation has consistently been demonstrated in histologic examinations of animal as well as human sinus mucosa biopsies, major physiologic adaptations have been observed, involving lack of glands in the lamina propria and increase in goblet cells (Bravetti et al. 1998, Timmenga et al. 2003).

Increase in sinus membrane thickness that persisted for more than 6 months in the absence of clinical signs of pathology has been confirmed radiographically, sonographically as well as endoscopically in 6% to 9% of augmented maxillary sinuses (Wiltfang et al. 2000, Ludwig et al. 2002). Sinus membrane thickening has equally been observed in 61% of implants protruding more than 4 mm into the maxillary sinus cavity (as seen in computed tomographic scans) without clinical signs of sinus infection 6 to

10 months after implant placement (Jung et al. 2007). Increased sinus membrane thickness can thus not be regarded radiologic evidence of chronic maxillary sinusitis (Kurien et al. 1989), however, it may rather indicate morphological alterations of the maxillary sinus membrane that must be suspected to impair the physiologic mucociliary activity of the mucosal lining of the maxillary sinus (Guo et al. 1998, Sul et al. 2008).

6.2. Bone Regeneration – Material and Methods

The aim of the following study was to evaluate bone regeneration after transcrestal maxillary sinus floor augmentation in a prospective clinical trial (Pommer et al. 2013b).

A total of 34 sinuses (15 left sinuses, 19 right sinuses) in 25 patients (13 men, 12 women, mean age of 45.6 ± 12.0 years) with deficient posterior maxillary ridges due to post-extraction sinus pneumatization were included. A detailed description of study medthodology is presented in chapter 3.2. In short, flapless transcrestal sinsus floor elevation was performed using the gel-pressure technique (Pommer & Watzek 2009). Following maxillary sinus membrane elevation a bone graft paste of synthetic nanoparticulate hydroxyapatite (Busenlechner et al. 2009) was injected underneath the maxillary sinus membrane and simultaneous implants were placed and sealed the transcrestal osteotomy. After transmucosal implant healing of 4 to 6 months, fixed partial dentures (single crowns or fixed bridges) were manufactured. CT scans were obtained prior to augmentation surgery, 1 week after, and 4 months after sinus membrane elevation surgery (Figure 6.1).

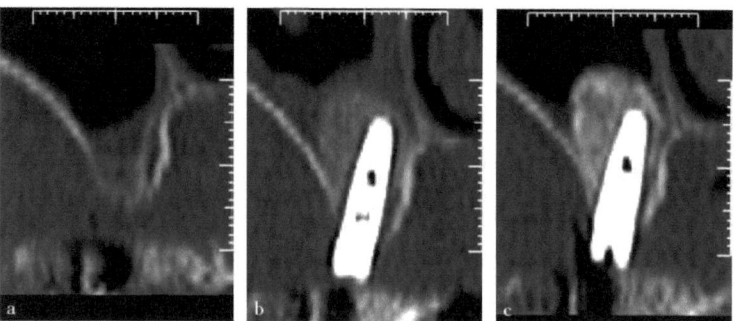

Figure 6.1: Cross-sectional computed tomographic cans (a) prior to surgery, (b) one week and (c) 4 months after transcrestal sinus floor augmentation.

Postoperative augmentation height was compared to bone height after the healing time of 4 months and mean vertical graft shrinkage was computed. Average radiographic bone density was measured in Hounsfield Units (HU) for every axial slice in a distance of 1 mm. Measurements were performed using the Easy Vision Workstation (Philips, Eindhoven, the Netherlands). All calculations were performed using R-project statistical software (R Foundation for Statistical Computing, Vienna, Austria).

6.3. Bone Regeneration – Study Results

Postoperative complications included transient maxillary sinusitis in four cases (11.8%) and two cases of graft sequestration which necessitated endoscopic removal (5.8%). The mean height of the augmented area was 11.2 ± 2.7 mm resulting in a mean postoperative height of 16.3 ± 2.8 mm.

After 4 months of graft healing the mean bone height was 16.2 ± 2.8 mm (mean vertical graft shrinkage: 0.1 mm). Graft shrinkage amounted to 1 mm (9.7%) in three cases and to 0.5 mm (6.5%) in two. Radiologic bone density after four months of healing was significantly higher in the first 7 mm adjacent to the former sinus floor (mean hounsfield units: 423) than in the more cranial part of the bone graft (mean hounsfield units: 372, p=0.006). This may indicate that bone grafts larger than 7 mm in height are not completely ossified after 4 months of healing.

6.4. Impact on Sinus Physiology – Material and Methods

The aim of the following study was to investigate the effect of sinus membrane elevation and bone augmentation of the maxillary sinus floor on sinus membrane thickness by within-subject comparison of pre- vs. post-augmentation computed tomographic scans (Pommer et al. 2012a).

Thirty-five patients with a mean age of 54.7 ± 10.2 years (range: 27-69 years) underwent sinus floor augmentation via a lateral approach (bony window in the facial wall of the maxillary sinus) at the Department of Oral Surgery (Bernhard Gottlieb School of Dentistry, Vienna Medical University, Austria) in the years 2006 to 2007. Out of the 21 female and 14 male patients, 4 (11.4%) were smokers. Patients presented with partially edentulous (5 patients) or completely edentulous (30 patients) maxillae that did not allow simultaneous implant placement at the time of augmentation surgery. Following inclusion criteria were applied: [1] residual alveolar ridge height of less than 4 mm, [2] absence of any signs of maxillary sinus pathology prior to as well as following maxillary sinus floor augmentation surgery, and [3] no interoperative evidence of iatrogenic perforation of the maxillary sinus membrane. Evaluation of a total of 65 sinus floor augmentation procedures using 50% autologous bone grafted from the hip and 50% deproteinized bovine bone material (Bio-Oss®, Geistlich, Wolhusen, Switzerland) was performed. A total of 13 sinus floor augmentation procedures were excluded due to sinus membrane perforation (inclusion criterium 3) resulting in a membrane perforation rate of 13%. In partially edentulous patients, the contralateral non-augmented sinuses served as negative controls. Computed tomographic scans were performed 1 to 6 months prior to sinus floor elevation (preoperative CT) as well as 4 to 6 months after sinus augmentation surgery (postoperative CT) prior to implant insertion. The study was approved by the local ethics committee (EK 219/2009) and all patients gave their informed consent to radiologic examination and scientific use of data.

Preoperative as well as postoperative computed tomographic scans were acquired with the same conventional CT scanner (Tomoscan SR-6000, Philips, Eindhoven, the Netherlands) using a standard dental CT investigation protocol (1.5 mm slice thickness, 120 kV, 2s scan time, 75 mA, 1.0 mm table feed, high-resolution bone filter, 100 to 120 mm field of view) for all the patients (Gahleitner et al. 2003). Measurements were performed at two axial CT slices, 15 and 20 mm above the alveolar crest, of the preoperative and postoperative scans, respectively (Figure 6.2), on the Easy Vision Workstation (Software Release 2.1, Philips, Eindhofen, the Netherlands).

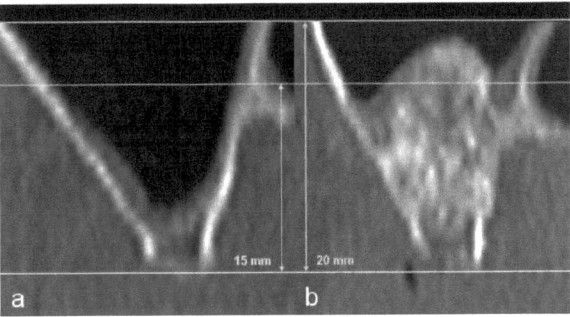

Figure 6.2: Computed tomographic cross-sections indicating the height of axial slices used for measurement: 15 mm (yellow) and 20 mm (turquoise) above the alveolar crest of the preoperative (a) as well as postoperative (b) scans, respectively.

By the use of Hounsfield-threshold analysis and affinity-based image segmentation (Veldkamp et al. 2010), the following measurements were taken on the preoperative CT scans (Figure 6.3a): perimeter (A) and area (B) of the sinus bone as well as pneumatized area (C) of the sinus cavity. Measurements on the postoperative scans additionally included perimeter (D) and area (E) of the bone graft (Figure 6.3b). Total bone height following graft healing and residual alveolar ridge height prior to augmentation surgery were assessed on cross sections at the position of the maximum apico-coronal extension of the bone graft.

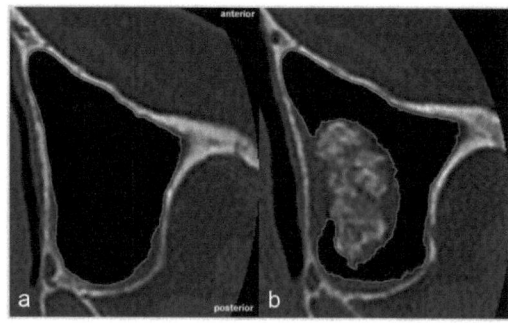

Figure 6.3: Preoperative (a) and postoperative (b) axial CT slices 15 mm above the alveolar crest (corresponding to the yellow line in Figure 6.2). Parts of the nasal cavity appear on the left side, the zygomatic arch on the right side in (a) and (b), while bone graft material (outlined in red) can only be seen in the postoperative CT (b) and is surrounded by the pneumatized sinus cavity on the anterior, lateral and posterior aspect. Measurements involved area and perimeter of the sinus bone (blue outline), pneumatized area of the sinus cavity (green outline), as well as area and perimeter of the bone graft material (red outline).

Thickness values of the maxillary sinus membrane were calculated by $t_1=(B-C)/A$ on the preoperative CTs, while postoperative sinus membrane thickness was computed by $t_2=(B-C-E)/(A+D)$ using average determination of the sinus membrane area per sinus perimeter. Postoperative increase in membrane thickness is thus represented by positive values of $\Delta t = t_2 - t_1$. Descriptive statistic analyses involved mean and standard deviation (given normal distribution of all data). Within-subject comparison (preoperative vs. postoperative conditions) was performed using paired t-tests at a significance level of $p<0.05$. Pearson's correlation coefficient (Williams

1996) was used to investigate associations between corresponding axial slices of preoperative and postoperative scans, as well as between Δt and relevant baseline variables (patient age, preoperative residual ridge height and postoperative total bone graft height). The results of the two axial computed tomographic slices in each sinus (15 and 20 mm above the alveolar crest, respectively) were plotted in these analyses (given no statistical significant difference, p<0.05). All calculations were performed using R-project statistical software (R Foundation for Statistical Computing, Vienna, Austria).

6.5. Impact on Sinus Physiology – Study Results

Preoperative and postoperative computed tomographic scans demonstrated high levels of reproducibility (r=0.97, p<0.001) of the corresponding axial alices, promoting accuracy of comparison (Gahleitner et al. 2008). No significant differences prior vs. following sinus augmentation surgery were seen regarding sinus perimeter (A) and sinus area (B) measurements (Table 6.1) showing a mean deviation of 7.5% (p<0.05). Repeated measurements yielded low levels of intra-observer variability (due to automated image segmentation) with deviations smaller than 1% on average. Non-augmented sinuses in partially edentulous patients (negative controls) revealed no statistically significant difference in maxillary sinus membrane thickness between the two (preoperative vs. postoperative) computed tomographic scans (p=0.321): postoperative increase in sinus membrane thickness of 0.03 mm could be observed in only 1 control sinus, while the remainder (80%) did not show any evidence of sinus membrane thickening. Mean residual alveolar ridge height prior to bone augmentation measured 2.1 ± 0.9 mm. Mean preoperative maxillary sinus membrane thickness (t_1)

measured 0.8 ± 1.2 mm, ranging from 0.0 mm to a maximum of 4.7 mm and showing no significant difference between measurements on the two axial CT slices, 15 and 20 mm above the alveolar crest (p=0.062). Higher values of preoperative sinus membrane thickness were detected in smokers (1.3 ± 1.4 mm) compared to non-smokers (0.7 ± 1.1 mm), the difference, however, did not reach statistical significance (p=0.191).

	preoperative CT scan		postoperative CT scan	
	axial slice 15 mm supracrestal	axial slice 20 mm supracrestal	axial slice 15 mm supracrestal	axial slice 20 mm supracrestal
A=perimeter (mm)	89.0 ± 12.1	96.9 ± 15.7	94.4 ± 13.5	102.7 ± 13.7
B=sinus area (mm^2)	445.7 ± 112.9	539.1 ± 114.3	497.0 ± 120.9	584.6 ± 127.8
C=pneumatized area (mm^2)	356.9 ± 145.8	483.5 ± 155.3	308.4 ± 148.6	383.3 ± 209.1
D=graft perimeter (mm)	-	-	46.8 ± 22.8	14.2 ± 21.5
E=graft area (mm^2)	-	-	156.4 ± 111.1	35.8 ± 66.8
t=membrane thickness (mm)	1.0 ± 1.4	0.6 ± 1.1	1.4 ± 1.1	1.7 ± 1.8

Table 6.1: Measurements on preoperative and postoperative computed tomographic scans (A-E) and computed maxillary sinus membrane thickness (mean ± standard deviation).

Mean thickess of the maxillary sinus membrane on the postoperative CT scans (t_2) measured 1.5 ± 1.3 mm without significant differences between the two axial slices, 15 and 20 mm above the alveolar crest (p=0.124).

Within-subject comparison revealed significantly higher values of sinus membrane thickness following augmentation surgery compared to preoperative conditions (p<0.001). The mean increase in membrane thickness measured 0.8 ± 1.6 mm. No increase in sinus membrane thickness could be seen in 18 maxillary sinuses (28%). The remainder 47 sinuses (72%) demonstrated thickening of the maxillary sinus membrane following bone augmentation surgery of 1.4 ± 1.2 mm on average. The maximum increase in sinus membrane thickness was 4.4 mm (Figure 6.4).

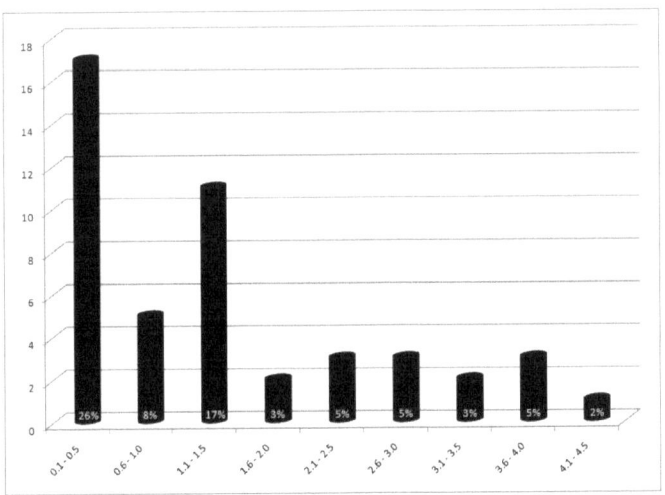

Figure 6.4: Absolute and relative frequencies (%) of sinus membrane thickening following maxillary sinus floor augmentation (maximum: 4.4 mm) according to groups of 0.5 mm.

Post-augmentation bone height averaged 14.4 ± 3.8 mm and did not show linear correlation to postoperative membrane thickenung (r=0.241), neither did preoperative residual alveolar ridge height (r=0.079) and patient age (r=0.242). Postoperative values of maxillary sinus membrane thickness were significantly higher (p=0.007) in smokers (2.7 ± 1.5 mm) compared to non-smokers (1.4 ± 1.2 mm), yet, sinus membrane thickening (Δt) as a result of sinus augmentation surgery did not show significant differences (p=0.228) between smoking patients (mean thickness increase: 1.4 ± 1.5 mm) compared to non-smokers (mean thickness increase: 0.7 ± 1.5 mm). Membrane reaction in maxillary sinuses that already showed above average thickness values prior to surgery (i.e. preoperative membrane thickness greater than 0.8 mm in a total of 19 sinuses) did not show any significant differences regarding neither sinus membrane thickness increase (p=0.070) nor mean postoperative values of maxillary sinus membrane thickness (p=0.260).

6.6. Discussion

The results of the present investigation on the effect of maxillary sinus floor augmentation on sinus physiology (Pommer et al. 2012a) reveal that sinus membrane thickness differs significantly prior to (0.8 ± 1.2 mm) vs. after (1.5 ± 1.3 mm) augmentation surgery (p<0.001) demonstrating mean values of thickness increase of 0.8 ± 1.6 mm (maximum: 4.4 mm). Preoperative radiographic membrane thickness was in line with average physiologic values of up to 1 mm reported in study that measured maxillary sinus membrane thickness in a clinical setting (Morgensen & Tos 1977, Aimetti et al. 2008, Pommer et al. 2009). No changes in membrane thickness could be seen in non-augmented sinuses, the control group of the present study, however, comprised only 5 sinuses of patients with partially edentulous maxillae as it seemed unethical to subject untreated patients to computed tomographic imaging in dublicate. Seventy-two percent of sinuses, by contrast, demonstrated thickening of the maxillary sinus membrane following bone graft surgery with a mean increase of 1.4 mm (maximum: 4.4 mm). A case series reporting on maxillary sinus membrane thickening found a considerably lower frequency of 4% in computed tomographies 8 to 10 months after maxillary sinus floor augmentation (Peleg et al. 1999). However, these measurements may not be comparable to the present results obtained by the use of three-dimensional automated Hounsfield-threshold-based CT evaluation, as they represent maximum values of sinus membrane thickness recorded at 5 borders of the bone graft area (apical, buccal, palatal, mesial, buccal). The limitations of conventional two-dimensional radiographic methods to measure changes in sinus membrane thickness as small as 1.4 mm, on average, may also serve as an explanation for the low rate of maxillary sinus membrane thickening of 6% to 9% identified by Waters' view x-rays following sinus bone augmentation (Wiltfang et al. 2000, Ludwig et al. 2002).

Bone graft materials used for maxillary sinus floor augmentation may as well have a significant impact on sinus membrane reactions. A mixture of autogenous bone harvested from an extraoral donor site in combination with deproteinized bovine bone substitute material was used in the present investigation. Major histological modifications of the maxillary sinus membrane were observed in both groups when a resorbable bone substitute material was used exclusively as well as in combination with autogenous bone grafts in a goat model (Bravetti et al. 1998). These modifications involved increase in the number of goblet cells and, on the other hand, decreased numbers of both ciliated cells as well as glands in the lamina propria and have been interpreted as adaptive reaction to bone graft surgery highly likely to result in significantly altered composition of the produced sinus mucus (Timmenga et al. 2003, Pignataro et al. 2008). In a dog model, by contrast, no ultrastructural alterations could be found after maxillary sinus membrane elevation and simultaneous placement of dental implants without the use of any bone (substitute) materials (Sul et al. 2008). As exclusively non-human primates present with maxillary sinus shape and size comparable to humans as well as similar rates of bone metabolism, animal models may have significant limitations, however (Margolin et al. 1998, McAllister et al. 1999). Tissue response to heterograft and allograft materials in the only human autopsy report to date showed lack of chronic inflammatory reaction but did not provide details on the impact of sinus bone grafts on maxillary sinus membrane physiology (Whittaker et al. 1989).

Furthermore, differences between sinus floor elevation via a lateral approach (Boyne & James 1980) and transcrestal elevation techniques (Summers 1994) may exist. Mucociliary impairment in the region of the maxillary sinus floor may only mildly disturb overall mucociliary clearance (Bravetti et al. 1998), however, the effects of transcrestal sinus floor augmentation on sinus physiology has not been investigated to date. Intraoperative endoscopy during sinus membrane elevation via a lateral approach confirmed that mucociliary function terminates in the elevated areas of the membrane (Griffa et al. 2010), while it remains hard to predict what kind of reactions to the surgical trauma of membrane elevation have to be expected in long-term (Pignataro et al. 2008). Perforation of the maxillary sinus membrane is caused by elevation forces that exceed the load limits of the membrane (Pommer & Watzek 2009). Morphologic regeneration of the sinus membrane has been shown to occur within 12 weeks after injury according to experimental research, while full functional recovery of its mucociliary activity may take significantly longer than that (Kim et al. 2008). Defect healing of torn sinus membranes is likely to result in scar tissue formation and significant impairment of mucociliary function even though resorbable membranes can be successfully used in 95% of cases to repair iatrogenic perforations during sinus membrane elevation (Schwartz-Arad et al. 2004).

The main factor in preserving sinus physiology is mucociliary clearance. It requires both normal ciliary structure and regular ciliary function (Kim et al. 2008). Defective ciliary function may lead to impairment of mucociliary transport even though the number of cilia may be normal (Guo et al. 1998). Assessment of the ciliary beat frequency (CBF) has been regarded as an indicator for effective movement of the cilia. Even physiologic CBF values (10 to 20 Hz), however, do not guarantee proper function (Abdel-Hak et al. 1998). In addition to regular CBF values, ciliary wave disorder (CWD), i.e. the degree of variation in the beat direction of individual cilia, has to be considered. High values of CWD, similar to low values of CBF, can also cause impairment of mucociliary clearance (Kim et al. 2008). There are three endoscopic methods to assess rates of mucociliary clearance quantitatively: the saccharine time test, the India ink test and radioisotopic testing (Asai et al. 2000, Toskala & Rautiainen 2005). To date, however, none of these three test have ever been performed in the grafted maxillary sinus.

Within the limits of the present radiologic study it can be concluded that significant variability of sinus membrane response to augmentation of the maxillary sinus floor can be observed. The majority of cases demonstrated radiographic thickening of the maxillary sinus membrane – even in asymptomatic clinical conditions – indicating morphological alterations in reaction to sinus augmentation surgery, while no ecidence of membrane reactions was found in 28% of sinuses. These findings may, however, not be extrapolated to long-term outcomes, so it should be kept in midn that they relate to a follow-up period of 4 to 6 months after bone grafting. It needs to be clarified whether the observed effects are transient or persistent in nature. Further studies are also needed to evaluate the impact of bone augmentation material, surgical approach as well as presence and extent of iatrogenic perforations of the maxillary sinus membrane and to investiagte the physiologic impact of transcrestal sinus floor elevation on mucociliary clearance of the maxillary sinus.

7. CONCLUSIONS

- The use of fluid- or gel-pressure carries the potential of reducing the risk of maxillary sinus membrane perforation in minimally invasive transcrestal sinus membrane elevation. The maximum height of membrane elevation was 10.6 mm on average and better results can be expected compared to osteotome-mediated elevation, due to the even distribution of elevation forces. Higher membrane elevation can be acchieved in narrow sinuses showing a small angle between the buccal and palatal sinus wall.

- No significant differences regarding the risk of maxillary sinus membrane perforation could be found between transcrestal sinus osteotomy using drills with rounded tips and internal irrigation compared to sinus floor infracture using osteotomes in a prospective clinical trial. Cut selectivity of alternative techniques such as piezoelectric devices or laser osteotomy may help to further reduce membrane perforation rates.

- Perforation of the maxillary sinus membrane (mean thickness: 90 µm) can be expected to occurr at a mean tension of 7.3 N/mm². The membrane can be stretchend to 125% of its original size on average, while thicker membranes demonstrate significantly higher load limits. The Schneiderian membrane's mean modulus of elasticity is 0.058 GPa and the mean force of membrane adhesion to the bony sinus floor is 0.05 N/mm. These data allow for three-dimensional dynamic finite element analyses to estimate maximum height of sinus membrane elevation that can safely be acchieved, as well as amount of graft material required, already prior to augmentation surgery. Moreover, simulation of the three-dimensional pattern of maxillary sinus membrane elevation may be performed in complex cases of multiple transcrestal osteotomies or the presence of maxillary sinus septa.

- Sinus septa can be found in 29% of maxillary sinuses on average. Septa prevalence is significantly higher in edentulous compared to dentate ridges. While bilateral septa can be found in 17% of patients, multiple septa per sinus occur only in 4%. The majority (55%) are located in first and second molar regions and 88% show a transverse (buccopalatal) orientation. Their mean height measures 7.5 mm. Septa diagnosis using panoramic radiographs yield incorrect results in 29% of cases.

- Primary stability of dental implants placed in conjunction with transcrestal sinus floor augmentation seems to be determined primarily by bone quality of the sinus floor while no significant impact of residual alveolar ridge height or implant diameter could be found. Preoperative bone density measurement in computed tomographies may thus provide helpful information to avoid lack of sufficient primary stability of simultaneous implants in one-stage transcrestal sinus floor elevation.

- Significant radiologic thickening of the maxillary sinus membrane 4 to 6 months after sinus floor elevation would suggest that the sinus membrane undergoes morphological modifications as a reaction to bone grafting even in healthy clinical conditions. Future research on the effect of transcrestal sinus floor elevation on maxillary sinus physiology and mucociliary clearance is needed.

- Bone regeneration following transcrestal sinus membrane elevation (mean augmentation height: 11.2 mm, mean vertical graft shrinkage: 0.1 mm) was generally uneventful while transient maxillary sinusitis could be seen in 12%. Bone density measurements indicate that bone grafts larger than 7 mm in height had not completely undergone ossification at 4 months after augmentation surgery.

8. REFERENCES

Abdel-Hak B, Gunkel A, Kanonier G, Schrott-Fischer A, Ulmer H & Thumfart W (1998) Ciliary beat frequency, olfaction and endoscopic sinus surgery. *ORL J Otorhinolaryngol Relat Spec* 60:202-205.

Agrawal S, Agrawal J & Agrawal TP (2005) Use of trypan blue to confirm the patency of filtering surgery. *J Cataract Refract Surg* 31:235-237.

Aimetti M, Massei G, Morra M, Cardesi E & Romano F (2008) Correlation between gingival phenotype and Schneiderian membrane thickness. *Int J Oral Maxillofac Implants* 23:1128-1132.

Akça K, Chang TL, Tekdemir I & Fanuscu MI (2006) Biomechanical aspects of initial intraosseous stability and implant design: a quantitative micro-morphometric analysis. *Clin Oral Implants Res* 17:465-472.

Ardekian L, Oved-Peleg E, Mactei EE & Peled M (2006) The clinical significance of sinus membrane perforation during augmentation of the maxillary sinus. *J Oral Maxillofac Surg* 64:277-282.

Ariji Y, Kuroki T, Moriguchi S, Ariji E & Kanda S (1994) Age changes in the volume of the human maxillary sinus: a study using computed tomography. *Dentomaxillofac Radiol* 23:163-168.

Asai K, Haruna S, Otori N, Yanagi K, Fukami M & Moriyama H (2000) Saccharin test of maxillary sinus mucociliary function after endoscopic sinus surgery. *Laryngoscope* 110:117-122.

Att W, Bernhart J & Strub JR (2009) Fixed rehabilitation of the edentulous maxilla: possibilities and clinical outcome. *J Oral Maxillofac Surg* 67:60-73.

Aust R & Drettner B (1974) The functional size of the human maxillary ostium in vivo. *Acta Otolaryngol* 78:432-435.

Aust R, Bäcklund L, Drettner B, Falck B & Jung B (1978) Comparative measurements of the mucosal blood flow in the human maxillary sinus by plethysmography and by xenon. *Acta Otolaryngol* 85:111-115.

Barone A, Santini S, Marconcini S, Giacomelli L, Gherlone E & Covani U (2008) Osteotomy and membrane elevation during the maxillary sinus augmentation procedure. A comparative study: piezoelectric device vs. conventional rotative instruments. *Clin Oral Implants Res* 19:511-515.

Berengo M, Sivolella S, Majzoub Z & Cordioli G (2004) Endoscopic evaluation of the bone-added osteotome sinus floor elevation procedure. *Int J Oral Maxillofac Surg* 33:189-194.

Betts NJ & Miloro M (1994) Modification of the sinus lift procedure for septa in the maxillary antrum. *J Oral Maxillofac Surg* 52:332-333.

Bischof JC & He X (2005) Thermal stability of proteins. *Ann N Y Acad Sci* 1066:12-33.

Blanton PL & Biggs NL (1969) Eighteen hundred years of controversy: the paranasal sinuses. *Am J Anat* 124:135-147.

Bolger WE, Woodruff WW Jr, Morehead J & Parsons DS (1990) Maxillary sinus hypoplasia: classification and description of associated uncinate process hypoplasia. *Otolaryngol Head Neck Surg* 103:759-765.

Borris TJ & Weber CR (1998) Intraoperative nasal transillumination for maxillary sinus augmentation procedures: a technical note. *Int J Oral Maxillofac Implants* 13:569-570.

Boyne PJ & James RA (1980) Grafting of the maxillary sinus floor with autogenous marrow and bone. *J Oral Surg* 38:613-616.

Bravetti P, Membre H, Marchal L & Jankowski R (1998) Histologic changes in the sinus membrane after maxillary sinus augmentation in goats. *J Oral Maxillofac Surg* 56:1170-1176.

Brook I (1981) Aerobic and anaerobic bacterial flora of normal maxillary sinuses. *Laryngoscope* 91:372-376.

Busenlechner D, Huber CD, Vasak C, Dobsak A, Gruber R & Watzek G (2009) Sinus augmentation analysis revised: the gradient of graft consolidation. *Clin Oral Implants Res* 20:1078-1083.

Carothers DG, Graham SM, Jia HP, Ackermann MR, Tack BF & McCray PB Jr (2001) Production of beta-defensin antimicrobial peptides by maxillary sinus mucosa. *Am J Rhinol* 15:175-179.

Chanavaz M (1990) Maxillary sinus: anatomy, physiology, surgery, and bone grafting related to implantology - eleven years of surgical experience (1979-1990). *J Oral Implantol* 16:199-209.

Chen L & Cha J (2005) An 8-year retrospective study: 1,100 patients receiving 1,557 implants using the minimally invasive hydraulic sinus condensing technique. *J Periodontol* 76:482-491.

Chiapasco M, Zaniboni M & Boisco M (2006) Augmentation procedures for the rehabilitation of deficient edentulous ridges with oral implants. *Clin Oral Implants Res* 17(Suppl):136-159.

Chiriac G, Herten M, Schwarz F, Rothamel D & Becker J (2005) Autogenous bone chips: influence of a new piezoelectric device (Piezosurgery) on chip morphology, cell viability and differentiation. *J Clin Periodontol* 32:994-999.

Cho SC, Wallace SS, Froum SJ & Tarnow DP (2001) Influence of anatomy on Schneiderian membrane perforations during sinus elevation surgery: three-dimensional analysis. *Pract Proced Aesthet Dent* 13:160-163.

Chrcanovic BR & Freire-Maia B (2010) Maxillary sinus aplasia. *Oral Maxillofac Surg* 14:187-191.

Chumbley LC, Morgan AM & Musallam I (1990) Hydroxypropyl methylcellulose in extracapsular cataract surgery with intraocular lens implantation: intraocular pressure and inflammatory response. *Eye* 4:121-126.

Cook HE & Haber J (1987) Bacteriology of the maxillary sinus. *J Oral Maxillofac Surg* 45:1011-1014.

Cosci F & Luccioli M (2000) A new sinus lift technique in conjunction with placement of 265 implants: a 6-year retrospective study. *Implant Dent* 9:363-368.

Dargaud J, Lamotte C, Dainotti JP & Morin A (2001) Venous drainage and innervation of the maxillary sinus. *Morphologie* 85:11-13.

das Neves FD, Fones D, Bernardes SR, do Prado CJ & Neto AJ (2006) Short implants - an analysis of longitudinal studies. *Int J Oral Maxillofac Implants* 21:86-93.

Dazert S, Mlynski R, Brors D, Sudhoff H & Prescher A (2004) Infection transfer between the maxillary sinus and endocranium. *HNO* 52:631-634.

De Leonardis D & Pecora GE (2000) Prospective study on the augmentation of the maxillary sinus with calcium sulfate: histological results. *J Periodontol* 71:940-947.

Del Fabbro M, Testori T, Francetti L & Weinstein R (2004) Systematic review of survival rates for implants placed in the grafted maxillary sinus. *Int J Periodontics Restorative Dent* 24:565-577.

Deppe H & Horch HH (2007) Laser applications in oral surgery and implant dentistry. *Lasers Med Sci* 22:217-221.

Drettner B & Aust R (1975) Investigation of the blood flow in the maxillary sinus. *Rhinology* 13:167-171.

Eisner G (1983) General considerations concerning viscous materials in ophthalmic surgery. *Trans Ophthalmol Soc UK* 103:247-253.

Elian N, Wallace S, Cho SC, Jalbout ZN & Froum S (2005) Distribution of the maxillary artery as it relates to sinus floor augmentation. *Int J Oral Maxillofac Implants* 20:784-787.

Ella B, Noble Rda C, Lauverjat Y, Sédarat C, Zwetyenga N, Siberchicot F & Caix P (2008) Septa within the sinus: effect on elevation of the sinus floor. *Br J Oral Maxillofac Surg* 46:464-467.

Emmerich D, Att W & Stappert C (2005) Sinus floor elevation using osteotomes: a systematic review and meta-analysis. *J Periodontol* 76:1237-1251.

Endo T, Abe R, Kuroki H, Kojima K, Oka K & Shimooka S (2010) Cephalometric evaluation of maxillary sinus sizes in different malocclusion classes. *Odontology* 98:65-72.

Engelke W & Capobianco M (2005) Flapless sinus floor augmentation using endoscopy combined with CT scan-designed surgical templates: method and report of 6 consecutive cases. *Int J Oral Maxillofac Implants* 20:891-897.

Engelke W & Deckwer I (1997) Endoscopically controlled sinus floor augmentation. A preliminary report. *Clin Oral Implants Res* 8:527-531.

Engelke W, Schwarzwäller W, Behnsen A & Jacobs HG (2003) Subantroscopic laterobasal sinus floor augmentation (SALSA): an up-to-5-year clinical study. *Int J Oral Maxillofac Implants* 18:135-143.

Falck B, Aust R, Svanholm H & Bäcklund L (1989) The effect of physical work on the mucosal blood flow and gas exchange in the human maxillary sinus. *Rhinology* 27:241-250.

Falck B, Svanholm H, Aust R & Bäcklund L (1990a) Blood flow and pulse amplitude in the mucosa of the human maxillary sinus in relation to body posture. *Rhinology* 28:169-176.

Falck B, Svanholm H & Aust R (1990b) The effect of Xylometazoline on the mucosa of human maxillary sinus. *Rhinology* 28:239-247.

Fenner M, Vairaktaris E, Fischer K, Schlegel KA, Neukam FW & Nkenke E (2009) Influence of residual alveolar bone height on osseointegration of implants in the maxilla: a pilot study. *Clin Oral Implants Res* 20:555-559.

Fernandes CL (2004) Forensic ethnic identification of crania: the role of the maxillary sinus - a new approach. *Am J Forensic Med Pathol* 25:302-313.

Ferrante SL, Schreiman JS, Rouse JW, Rysavy JA, Cheng SC & Frick MP (1990) Iopamidol as a gastrointestinal contrast agent. Lack of peritoneal reactivity. *Invest Radiol* 25:141-145.

Ferrigno N, Laureti M & Fanali S (2006) Dental implants placement in conjunction with osteotome sinus floor elevation: a 12-year life-table analysis from a prospective study on 588 ITI implants. *Clin Oral Implants Res* 17:194-205.

Flanagan D (2005) Arterial supply of maxillary sinus and potential for bleeding complication during lateral approach sinus elevation. *Implant Dent* 14:336-338.

Fleming TC, Merrill DL & Girard LJ (1959) Studies of the irritating action of methylcellulose. *AMA Arch Ophthalmol* 61:565-567.

Fortin T, Camby E, Alik M, Isidori M & Bouchet H (2011) Panoramic Images versus Three-Dimensional Planning Software for Oral Implant Planning in Atrophied Posterior Maxillary: A Clinical Radiological Study. *Clin Implant Dent Relat Res* [Epub ahead of print]

Gahleitner A, Watzek G & Imhof H (2003) Dental CT: imaging technique, anatomy, and pathologic conditions of the jaws. *Eur Radiol* 13:366-376.

Gahleitner A, Kuchler U, Homolka P, Heschl J, Watzek G & Imhof H (2008) High-resolution CT of transplanted teeth: imaging technique and measurement accuracy. *Eur Radiol* 18:2975-2980.

Gannon PJ, Doyle WJ, Ganjian E, Marquez S, Gnoy A, Gabrielle HS & Lawson W (1997) Maxillary sinus mucosal blood flow during nasal vs tracheal respiration. *Arch Otolaryngol Head Neck Surg* 123:1336-1340.

González-Santana H, Peñarrocha-Diago M, Guarinos-Carbó J & Sorní-Bröker M (2007) A study of the septa in the maxillary sinuses and the subantral alveolar processes in 30 patients. *J Oral Implantol* 33:340-343.

Gosau M, Rink D, Driemel O & Draenert FG (2009) Maxillary sinus anatomy: a cadaveric study with clinical implications. *Anat Rec (Hoboken)* 292:352-354.

Graf W & Martensson G (1957) Microscopical anatomy of the nerves in the lateral wall of the maxillary sinus. *Acta Otolaryngol* 47:114-122.

Griffa A, Berrone M, Boffano P, Viterbo S & Berrone S (2010) Mucociliary function during maxillary sinus floor elevation. *J Craniofac Surg* 21:1500-1502.

Guo Y, Majima Y, Hattori M, Seki S & Sakakura Y (1997) Effects of functional endoscopic sinus surgery on maxillary sinus mucosa. *Arch Otolaryngol Head Neck Surg* 123:1097-1100.

Guo Y, Majima Y, Hattori M, Seki S & Sakakura Y (1998) A comparative study of the ciliary area of the maxillary sinus mucosa and computed tomographic images. *Eur Arch Otorhinolaryngol* 255:202-204.

Güncü GN, Yildirim YD, Wang HL & Tözüm TF (2011) Location of posterior superior alveolar artery and evaluation of maxillary sinus anatomy with computerized tomography: a clinical study. *Clin Oral Implants Res* 22:1164-1167.

Haider R, Watzek G & Plenk H (1993) Effects of drill cooling and bone structure on IMZ implant fixation. *Int J Oral Maxillofac Implants* 8:83–91.

Hauman CH, Chandler NP & Tong DC (2002) Endodontic implications of the maxillary sinus: a review. *Int Endod J* 35:127-141.

Hernández-Alfaro F, Torradeflot MM & Marti C (2008) Prevalence and management of Schneiderian membrane perforations during sinus-lift procedures. *Clin Oral Implant Res* 19:91-98.

Hilton C, Wiedmann T, St Martin M, Humphrey B, Schleiffarth R & Rimell F (2008) Differential deposition of aerosols in the maxillary sinus of human cadavers by particle size. *Am J Rhinol* 22:395-398.

Hood CM, Schroter RC, Doorly DJ, Blenke EJ & Tolley NS (2009) Computational modeling of flow and gas exchange in models of the human maxillary sinus. *J Appl Physiol* 107:1195-1203.

Horton JE, Tarpley TM Jr & Wood LD (1975) The healing of surgical defects in alveolar bone produced with ultrasonic instrumentation, chisel, and rotary bur. *Oral Surg Oral Med Oral Pathol* 39:536-546.

Hosny M, Eldin SG & Hosny H (2002) Combined lidocaine 1% and hydroxypropyl methylcellulose 2.25% as a single anesthetic/viscoelastic agent in phacoemulsification. *J Cataract Refract Surg* 28:834-836.

Inanli S, Tutkun A, Batman C, Okar I, Uneri C & Sehitoglu MA (2000) The effect of endoscopic sinus surgery on mucociliary activity and healing of maxillary sinus mucosa. *Rhinology* 38:120-123.

Jovanovic S (2002) BIOLASE and UCLA successfully complete first Waterlase sinus surgery in the United States. *Dent Today* 21(8):27.

Jun BC, Song SW, Park CS, Lee DH, Cho KJ & Cho JH (2005) The analysis of maxillary sinus aeration according to aging process; volume assessment by 3-dimensional reconstruction by high-resolutional CT scanning. *Otolaryngol Head Neck Surg* 132:429-434.

Jung JH, Choi BH, Jeong SM, Li J, Lee SH & Lee HJ (2007) A retrospective study of the effects on sinus complications of exposing dental implants to the maxillary sinus cavity. *Oral Surg Oral Med Oral Pathol Oral Radiol Endod* 103:623-625.

Kalavagunta S & Reddy KT (2003) Extensive maxillary sinus pneumatization. *Rhinology* 41:113-117.

Karl M, Graef F, Heckmann S & Krafft T (2008) Parameters of resonance frequency measurement values: a retrospective study of 385 ITI dental implants. *Clin Oral Implants Res* 19:214-218.

Kasabah S, Slezák R, Simůnek A, Krug J & Lecaro MC (2002) Evaluation of the accuracy of panoramic radiograph in the definition of maxillary sinus septa. *Acta Medica (Hradec Kralove)* 45:173-175.

Kasabah S, Krug J, Simůnek A & Lecaro MC (2003) Can we predict maxillary sinus mucosa perforation? *Acta Medica (Hradec Králové)* 46:19-23.

Katranji A, Fotek P & Wang HL (2008) Sinus augmentation complications: etiology and treatment. *Implant Dentistry* 17:339-349.

Kesler G, Romanos G & Koren R (2006) Use of Er:YAG laser to improve osseointegration of titanium alloy implants - a comparison of bone healing. *Int J Oral Maxillofac Implants* 21:375-379.

Kfir E, Kfir V, Mijiritsky E, Rafaeloff R & Kaluski E (2006) Minimally invasive antral membrane balloon elevation followed by maxillary bone augmentation and implant fixation. *J Oral Implantol* 32:26-33.

Khoury F (1999) Augmentation of the sinus floor with mandibular bone block and simultaneous implantation: a 6-year clinical investigation. *Int J Oral Maxillofac Implants* 14:557-564.

Kim SG & Kim YK (2002) Use of a bone wax analogue to determine the amount of chin bone needed for sinus augmentation. *J Oral Maxillofac Surg* 60:600.

Kim HJ, Yoon HR, Kim KD, Kang MK, Kwak HH, Park HD, Han SH & Park CS (2003) Personal-computer-based three-dimensional reconstruction and simulation of maxillary sinus. *Surg Radiol Anat* 24:393-399.

Kim MJ, Jung UW, Kim CS, Kim KD, Choi SH, Kim CK & Cho KS (2006) Maxillary sinus septa: prevalence, height, location, and morphology. A reformatted computed tomography scan analysis. *J Periodontol* 77:903-908.

Kim YM, Lee CH, Won TB, Kim SW, Kim JW, Rhee CS & Min YG (2008) Functional recovery of rabbit maxillary sinus mucosa in two different experimental injury models. *Laryngoscope* 118:541-545.

Kimura Y, Yu DG, Fujita A, Yamashita A, Murakami Y & Matsumoto K (2001) Effects of erbium, chromium:YSGG laser irradiation on canine mandibular bone. *J Periodontol* 72:1178-1182.

Kirihene RK, Rees G & Wormald PJ (2002) The influence of the size of the maxillary sinus ostium on the nasal and sinus nitric oxide levels. *Am J Rhinol* 16:261-264.

Koymen R, Gocmen-Mas N, Karacayli U, Ortakoglu K, Ozen T & Yazici AC (2009) Anatomic evaluation of maxillary sinus septa: surgery and radiology. *Clin Anat* 22:563-570.

Krennmair G, Ulm C & Lugmayr H (1997) Maxillary sinus septa: incidence, morphology and clinical implications. *J Craniomaxillofac Surg* 25:261-265.

Krennmair G, Ulm C, Lugmayr H & Solar P (1999) The incidence, location, and height of maxillary sinus septa in the edentulous and dentate maxilla. *J Oral Maxillofac Surg* 57:667-671.

Kurien M, Raman R & Job A (1989) Roentgen examination of maxillary sinus, antral puncture and irrigation--a comparative study. *Singapore Med J* 30:565-567.

Lawson W, Patel ZM & Lin FY (2008) The development and pathologic processes that influence maxillary sinus pneumatization. *Anat Rec (Hoboken)* 291:1554-1563.

Lee WJ, Lee SJ & Kim HS (2010) Analysis of location and prevalence of maxillary sinus septa. *J Periodontal Implant Sci* 40:56-60.

Leopold D, Zinreich SJ, Simon BA, Cullen MM & Marcucci C (2000) Xenon-enhanced computed tomography quantifies normal maxillary sinus ventilation. *Otolaryngol Head Neck Surg* 122:422-424.

Li Y, Yang M, Fang Z, Du Z & Zhao W (2002) Microcirculation evaluation of the maxillary sinus mucosa in patients with chronic sinusitis. *Lin Chuang Er Bi Yan Hou Ke Za Zhi* 16:579-580.

Liesegang TJ, Bourne WM & Ilstrup DM (1986) The use of hydroxypropyl methylcellulose in extracapsular cataract extraction with intraocular lens implantation. *Am J Ophthalmol* 102:723-726.

Ludwig A, Merten HA, Wiltfang J, Engelke W & Wiese KG (2002) Evaluation of B-scan ultrasound, 3-D ultrasound, roentgen diagnosis and sinus endoscopy in follow-up assessment of the maxillary sinus after sinus floor elevation. *Mund Kiefer Gesichtschir* 6:341-345.

Lugmayr H, Krennmair G & Holzer H (1996) The morphology and incidence of maxillary sinus septa. *RöFo* 165:452-454.

Lund VJ (1988) The maxillary sinus in the higher primates. *Acta Otolaryngol* 105:163-171.

Lundgren S, Moy P, Johansson C & Nilsson H (1996) Augmentation of the maxillary sinus floor with particulated mandible: a histologic and histomorphometric study. *Int J Oral Maxillofac Implants* 11:760-766.

Maestre-Ferrín L, Galán-Gil S, Rubio-Serrano M, Peñarrocha-Diago M & Peñarrocha-Oltra D (2010) Maxillary sinus septa: a systematic review. *Med Oral* 15:e383-386.

Maestre-Ferrín L, Carrillo-García C, Galán-Gil S, Peñarrocha-Diago M & Peñarrocha-Diago M (2011) Prevalence, location, and size of maxillary sinus septa: panoramic radiograph versus computed tomography scan. *J Oral Maxillofac Surg* 69:507-511.

Marchack CB & Moy PK (2003) The use of a custom template for immediate loading with the definitive prosthesis: a clinical report. *J Calif Dent Assoc* 31:925-929.

Margolin MD, Cogan AG, Taylor M, Buck D, McAllister TN, Toth C & McAllister BS (1998) Maxillary sinus augmentation in the non-human primate: a comparative radiographic and histologic study between recombinant human osteogenic protein-1 and natural bone mineral. *J Periodontol* 69:911-919.

Mathew AL, Pai KM & Sholapurkar AA (2009) Maxillary sinus findings in the elderly: a panoramic radiographic study. *J Contemp Dent Pract* 10:e41-48.

Mazo Z, Peleg M & Gross M (1999) Sinus augmentation for single-tooth replacement in the posterior maxilla: a 3-year follow-up clinical report. *Int J Oral Maxillofac Implants* 14:55-60.

McAllister BS, Margolin MD, Cogan AG, Buck D, Hollinger JO & Lynch SE (1999) Eighteen-month radiographic and histologic evaluation of sinus grafting with anorganic bovine bone in the chimpanzee. *Int J Oral Maxillofac Implants* 14:361-368.

Meyers RM & Valvassori G (1998) Interpretation of anatomic variations of computed tomography scans of the sinuses: a surgeon's perspective. *Laryngoscope* 108:422-425.

Mikula SK, Gannon PJ, Shapiro J & Lawson W (1996) Gaseous dynamics of the rabbit maxillary sinus. *Laryngoscope* 106:152-155.

Morgensen C & Tos M (1977) Quantitative histology of the maxillary sinus. *Rhinology* 15:129-134.

Murakami G, Ohtsuka K, Sato I, Moriyama H, Shimada K & Tomita H (1994) The superior alveolar nerves: their topographical relationship and distribution to the maxillary sinus in human adults. *Okajimas Folia Anat Jpn* 70:319-328.

Müsebeck K & Rosenberg H (1978) Measurement of air flow in the maxillary sinus by hot-film technique. *Rhinology* 16:11-18.

Naitoh M, Suenaga Y, Kondo S, Gotoh K & Ariji E (2009) Assessment of maxillary sinus septa using cone-beam computed tomography: etiological consideration. *Clin Implant Dent Relat Res* 11:e52-58.

Naitoh M, Suenaga Y, Gotoh K, Ito M, Kondo S & Ariji E (2010) Observation of maxillary sinus septa and bony bridges using dry skulls between Hellman's dental age of IA and IIIC. *Okajimas Folia Anat Jpn* 87:41-47.

Nedir R, Bischof M, Briaux JM, Beyer S, Szmukler-Moncler S & Bernard JP (2004) A 7-year life table analysis from a prospective study on ITI implants with special emphasis on the use of short implants. Results from a private practice. *Clin Oral Implants Res* 15:150-157.

Nedir R, Bischof M, Vazquez L, Szmukler-Moncler S & Bernard JP (2006) Osteotome sinus floor elevation without grafting material: a 1-year prospective pilot study with ITI implants. *Clin Oral Implants Res* 17:679-686.

Neugebauer J, Ritter L, Mischkowski RA, Dreiseidler T, Scherer P, Ketterle M, Rothamel D & Zöller JE (2010) Evaluation of maxillary sinus anatomy by cone-beam CT prior to sinus floor elevation. *Int J Oral Maxillofac Implants* 25:258-265.

Nimigean V, Nimigean VR, Măru N, Sălăvăstru DI, Bădiţă D & Tuculină MJ (2008) The maxillary sinus floor in the oral implantology. *Rom J Morphol Embryol* 49:485-489.

Nkenke E, Schlegel A, Schultze-Mosgau S, Neukam FW & Wiltfang J (2002) The endoscopically controlled osteotome sinus floor elevation: a preliminary prospective study. *Int J Oral Maxillofac Implants* 17:557-566.

Noguerol B, Muñoz R, Mesa F, de Dios Luna J & O'Valle F (2006) Early implant failure. Prognostic capacity of Periotest: retrospective study of a large sample. *Clin Oral Implants Res* 17:459-464.

Oh HK & Rue SY (1998) Clinical anatomical study of maxillary sinus septum. *Korean J Oral Maxillofac Surg* 24:209.

O'Sullivan D, Sennerby L & Meredith N (2000) Measurements comparing the initial stability of five designs of dental implants: a human cadaver study. *Clin Implant Dent Relat Res* 2:85-92.

O'Sullivan D, Sennerby L, Jagger D & Meredith N (2004) A comparison of two methods of enhancing implant primary stability. *Clin Implant Dent Relat Res* 6:48-57.

Pang KP, Siow JK & Tan HM (2005) Migration of a foreign body in the maxillary sinus illustrating natural mucociliary action. *Med J Malaysia* 60:523-525.

Park YB, Jeon HS, Shim JS, Lee KW & Moon HS (2011) Analysis of the anatomy of the maxillary sinus septum using 3-dimensional computed tomography. *J Oral Maxillofac Surg* 69:1070-1078.

Peleg M, Chaushu G, Mazor Z, Ardekian L & Bakoon M (1999) Radiological findings of the post-sinus lift maxillary sinus: a computerized tomography follow-up. *J Periodontol* 70:1564-1573.

Perko D (1991) Temperature measurements in the maxillary sinus of rabbits. *Rhinology* 29:185-192.

Pignataro L, Mantovani M, Torretta S, Felisati G & Sambataro G (2008) ENT assessment in the integrated management of candidate for (maxillary) sinus lift. *Acta Otorhinolaryngol Ital* 28:110-119.

Pikos MA (1999) Maxillary sinus membrane repair: report of a technique for large perforations. *Implant Dent* 8:29-34.

Pjetursson BE, Tan WC, Zwahlen M & Lang NP (2009) A systematic review of the success of sinus floor elevation and survival of implants inserted in combination with sinus floor elevation. Part I: Lateral approach. *J Clin Perio* 35:216-240.

Pommer B & Watzek G (2009) Gel-pressure technique (GPT) for flapless transcrestal maxillary sinus floor elevation: a preliminary cadaveric study on a new surgical technique. *Int J Oral Maxillofac Implants* 24:817-822.

Pommer B, Unger E, Sütö D, Hack N & Watzek G (2009) Mechanical properties of the Schneiderian membrane in vitro. *Clin Oral Implants Res* 20:633-637.

Pommer B, Frantal S, Willer J, Posch M, Watzek G & Tepper G (2011) Impact of dental implant length on early failure rates: a meta-analysis of observational studies. *J Clin Periodontol* 38:856-863.

Pommer B, Dvorak G, Jesh P, Palmer RM, Watzek G & Gahleitner A (2012a) Effect of maxillary sinus floor augmentation on sinus membrane thickness in CT. *J Periodontol* 83:551-556.

Pommer B, Ulm C, Lorenzoni M, Palmer R, Watzek G & Zechner W (2012b) Prevalence, location and morphology of maxillary sinus septa: systematic review and meta-analysis. *J Clin Periodontol* 39:769-773.

Pommer B, Hof M, Fädler A, Gahleitner A, Watzek G & Watzak G (2012c) Primary implant stability in the sinus floor of atrophic human cadaver maxillae: impact of residual ridge height, bone density and implant diameter. *Clinical Oral Implants Research* [epub ahead of print]

Pommer B, Unger E, Schaller A, Zechner W & Watzek G (2013a) Maximum height of transcrestal maxillary sinus membrane elevation using osteotomes vs. liquid or gel pressure: computed tomography-based analyses. [under review]

Pommer B, Unger E & Watzek G (2013b) Transcrestal osteotomy for minimally invasive sinus floor elevation: a prospective clinical trial comparing drill- vs. osteotome-mediated techniques. [under review]

Pourzarandian A, Watanabe H, Aoki A, Ichinose S, Sasaki KM, Nitta H & Ishikawa I (2004) Histological and TEM examination of early stages of bone healing after Er:YAG laser irradiation. *Photomed Laser Surg* 22:342-350.

Privalov PL (1990) Cold denaturation of proteins. *Crit Rev Biochem Mol Biol* 25:281-305.

Qin Y & Li Z (1999) CT scanning analysis for maxillary sinus bony septum abnormalities and its clinical significance. *Lin Chuang Er Bi Yan Hou Ke Za Zhi* 13:53-55.

Reiser GM, Rabinovitz Z, Bruno J, Damoulis PD & Griffin TJ (2001) Evaluation of maxillary sinus membrane response following elevation with the crestal osteotome technique in human cadavers. *Int J Oral Maxillofac Implants* 16:833-840.

Robinson S & Wormald PJ (2005) Patterns of innervation of the anterior maxilla: a cadaver study with relevance to canine fossa puncture of the maxillary sinus. *Laryngoscope* 115:1785-1788.

Romanos GE, Gutknecht N, Dieter S, Schwarz F, Crespi R & Sculean A (2009) Laser wavelengths and oral implantology. *Lasers Med Sci* 24:961-970.

Roodenburg JLN, ten Bosch JJ & Borsboom PCF (1990) Measurement of the uniaxial elasticity of oral mucosa in vivo after CO_2-laser evaporation and surgical excision. *Int J Oral Maxillofac Surg* 19:181-183.

Rosano G, Taschieri S, Gaudy JF, Lesmes D & Del Fabbro M (2010) Maxillary sinus septa: a cadaveric study. *J Oral Maxillofac Surg* 68:1360-1364.

Rossetti PH, Bonachela WC & Rossetti LM (2010) Relevant anatomic and biomechanical studies for implant possibilities on the atrophic maxilla: critical appraisal and literature review. *J Prosthodont* 19:449-457.

Rysz M & Bakoń L (2009) Maxillary sinus anatomy variation and nasal cavity width: structural computed tomography imaging. *Folia Morphol (Warsz)* 68:260-264.

Sasaki KM, Aoki A, Ichinose S & Ishikawa I (2002) Ultrastructural analysis of bone tissue irradiated by Er:YAG Laser. *Lasers Surg Med* 31:322-332.

Scharf KE, Lawson W, Shapiro JM & Gannon PJ (1995) Pressure measurements in the normal and occluded rabbit maxillary sinus. *Laryngoscope* 105:570-574.

Schlee M, Steigmann M, Bratu E & Garg AK (2006) Piezosurgery: basics and possibilities. *Implant Dent* 15:334-340.

Schwartz-Arad D, Herzberg R & Dolev E (2004) The prevalence of surgical complications of the sinus graft procedure and their impact on implant survival. *J Periodontol* 75:511-516.

Schwarz F, Olivier W, Herten M, Sager M, Chaker A & Becker J (2007) Influence of implant bed preparation using an Er:YAG laser on the osseointegration of titanium implants: a histomorphometrical study in dogs. *J Oral Rehabil* 34:273-281.

Selcuk A, Ozcan KM, Akdogan O, Bilal N & Dere H (2008) Variations of maxillary sinus and accompanying anatomical and pathological structures. *J Craniofac Surg* 19:159-164.

Sharan A & Madjar D (2008) Maxillary sinus pneumatization following extractions: a radiographic study. *Int J Oral Maxillofac Implants* 23:48-56.

Shen EC, Fu E, Chiu TJ, Chang V, Chiang CY & Tu HP (2012) Prevalence and location of maxillary sinus septa in the Taiwanese population and relationship to the absence of molars. *Clin Oral Implants Res* 23:741-745.

Shibli JA, Faveri M, Ferrari DS, Melo L, Garcia RV, d'Avila S, Figueiredo LC & Feres M (2007) Prevalence of maxillary sinus septa in 1024 subjects with edentulous upper jaws: a retrospective study. *J Oral Implantol* 33:293-296.

Sirikçi A, Bayazit Y, Gümüsburun E, Bayram M & Kanlikana M (2000) A new approach to the classification of maxillary sinus hypoplasia with relevant clinical implications. *Surg Radiol Anat* 22:243-247.

Smith SG, Lindstrom RL, Miller RA, Hazel S, Skelnik D, Williams P & Mindrup E (1984) Safety and efficacy of 2% methylcellulose in cat and monkey cataract-implant surgery. *J Am Intraocul Implant Soc* 10:160-163.

Sohn DS, Lee JS, An KM & Romanos GE (2009) Erbium,chromium:yttrium-scandium-gallium-garnet laser-assisted sinus graft procedure. *Lasers Med Sci* 24:673-677.

Solar P, Geyerhofer U, Traxler H, Windisch A, Ulm C & Watzek G (1999) Blood supply to the maxillary sinus relevant to sinus floor elevation procedures. *Clin Oral Implants Res* 10:34-44.

Soltan M & Smiler DG (2005) Antral membrane balloon elevation. *J Oral Implantol* 31:85-90.

Sotirakis EG & Gonshor A (2005) Elevation of the maxillary sinus floor with hydraulic pressure. *J Oral Implantol* 31:197-204.

Stammberger H (1989). History of rhinology: anatomy of the paranasal sinuses. *Rhinology* 27:197-210.

Stellingsma C, Vissink A, Meijer HJ, Kuiper C & Raghoebar GM (2004) Implantology and the severely resorbed edentulous mandible. *Crit Rev Oral Biol Med* 15:240-248.

Stelzle F & Benner KU (2011) Evaluation of different methods of indirect sinus floor elevation for elevation heights of 10mm: an experimental ex vivo study. *Clin Implant Dent Relat Res* 13:124-133.

Stübinger S, Kuttenberger J, Filippi A, Sader R & Zeilhofer HF (2005) Intraoral piezosurgery: preliminary results of a new technique. *J Oral Maxillofac Surg* 63:1283-1287.

Stübinger S, Landes C, Seitz O, Zeilhofer HF & Sader R (2008) Ultrasonic bone cutting in oral surgery: a review of 60 cases. *Ultraschall Med* 29:66-71.

Stübinger S, Nuss K, Sebesteny T, Saldamli B, Sader R & von Rechenberg B (2010) Erbium-doped yttrium aluminium garnet laser-assisted access osteotomy for maxillary sinus elevation: a human and animal cadaver study. *Photomed Laser Surg* 28:39-44.

Suguimoto RM, Trindade IK & Carvalho RM (2006) The use of negative pressure for the sinus lift procedure: a technical note. *Int J Oral Maxillofac Implants* 21:455-458.

Sul SH, Choi BH, Li J, Jeong SM & Xuan F (2008) Histologic changes in the maxillary sinus membrane after sinus membrane elevation and the simultaneous insertion of dental implants without the use of grafting materials. *Oral Surg Oral Med Oral Pathol Oral Radiol Endod* 105:e1-e5.

Sullivan SM, Bulard RA, Meaders R & Patterson MK (1997) The use of fibrin adhesive in sinus lift procedures. *Oral Surg Oral Med Oral Pathol Oral Radiol Endod* 84:616-619.

Summers RB (1994) The osteotome technique. part 3 - less invasive methods of elevating the sinus floor. *Compend Contin Educ Dent* 15:698-708.

Sunukjian JR & DiFabio VE (1979) Barium outlining the maxillary sinus. *Oral Surg Oral Med Oral Pathol* 48:283.

Tan WC, Lang NP, Zwahlen M & Pjetursson BE (2008) A systematic review of the success of sinus floor elevation and survival of implants inserted in combination with sinus floor elevation. part II: transalveolar technique. *J Clin Perio* 35(Suppl):241-254.

Tawil G & Younan R (2003) Clinical evaluation of short, machined-surface implants followed for 12 to 92 months. *Int J Oral Maxillofac Implants* 18:894-901.

Taylor HA, Riley SE, Parks SE & Stevenson RE (1978) Long-term storage of tissue samples for cell culture. *In Vitro* 14:476-478.

ten Bruggenkate CM & van den Bergh JP (1998) Maxillary sinus floor elevation: a valuable pre-prosthetic procedure. *Periodontol 2000* 17:176-182.

Tepper G, Haas R, Schneider B, Watzak G, Mailath G, Jovanovic SA, Busenlechner D, Zechner W & Watzek G (2003) Effects of sinus lifting on voice quality. A prospective study and risk assessment. *Clin Oral Implants Res* 14:767-774.

Thor A, Sennerby L, Hirsch JM & Rasmusson L (2007) Bone formation at the maxillary sinus floor following simultaneous elevation of the mucosal lining and implant installation without graft material: an evaluation of 20 patients treated with 44 Astra Tech implants. *J Oral Maxillofac Surg* 65(Suppl 1):64-72.

Timmenga NM, Raghoebar GM, Liem RS, van Weissenbruch R, Manson WL & Vissink A (2003) Effects of maxillary sinus floor elevation surgery on maxillary sinus physiology. *Eur J Oral Sci* 111:189-197.

Tiwana PS, Kushner GM & Haug RH (2006) Maxillary sinus augmentation. *Dent Clin North Am* 50:409-424.

Toffler M (2004) Osteotome-mediated sinus floor elevation: a clinical report. *Int J Oral Maxillofac Implants* 19:266-273.

Tokushige E, Itoh K, Ushikai M, Katahira S & Fukuda K (1994) Localization of IL-1 beta mRNA and cell adhesion molecules in the maxillary sinus mucosa of patients with chronic sinusitis. *Laryngoscope* 104:1245-1250.

Toppozada HH & Talaat MA (1980) The normal human maxillary sinus mucosa. An electron microscopic study. *Acta Otolaryngol* 89:204-213.

Torrella F, Pitarch J, Cabanes G & Anitua E (1998) Ultrasonic ostectomy for the surgical approach of the maxillary sinus: a technical note. *Int J Oral Maxillofac Implants* 13:697-700.

Toscano NJ, Holtzclaw D & Rosen PS (2010) The effect of piezoelectric use on open sinus lift perforation: a retrospective evaluation of 56 consecutively treated cases from private practices. *J Periodontol* 81:167-171.

Toskala E & Rautiainen M (2005) Effects of surgery on the function of maxillary sinus mucosa. *Eur Arch Otorhinolaryngol* 262:236-240.

Traxler H, Windisch A, Geyerhofer U, Surd R, Solar P & Firbas W (1999) Arterial blood supply of the maxillary sinus. *Clin Anat* 12:417-421.

Uchida Y, Goto M, Katsuki T & Soejima Y (1998) Measurement of maxillary sinus volume using computerized tomographic images. *Int J Oral Maxillofac Implants* 13:811-818.

Ulm CW, Solar P, Krennmair G, Matejka M & Watzek G (1995) Incidence and suggested surgical management of septa in sinus-lift procedures. *Int J Oral Maxillofac Implants* 10:462-465.

Underwood AS (1910) An Inquiry into the Anatomy and Pathology of the Maxillary Sinus. *J Anat Physiol* 44:354-369.

Vallo J, Suominen-Taipale L, Huumonen S, Soikkonen K & Norblad A (2010) Prevalence of mucosal abnormalities of the maxillary sinus and their relationship to dental disease in panoramic radiography: results from the Health 2000 Health Examination Survey. *Oral Surg Oral Med Oral Pathol Oral Radiol Endod* 109:e80-87.

van den Bergh JP, ten Bruggenkate CM, Disch FJ & Tuinzing DB (2000) Anatomical aspects of sinus floor elevations. *Clin Oral Implants Res* 11:256-265.

van Steenberghe D, Naert I, Andersson M, Brajnovic I, Van Cleynenbreugel J & Suetens P (2002) A custom template and definitive prosthesis allowing immediate implant loading in the maxilla: A clinical report. *Int J Oral Maxillofac Implants* 17:663-670.

van Zyl AW & van Heerden WF (2009) A retrospective analysis of maxillary sinus septa on reformatted computerised tomography scans. *Clin Oral Implants Res* 20:1398-1401.

Velásquez-Plata D, Hovey LR, Peach CC & Alder ME (2002) Maxillary sinus septa: a 3-dimensional computerized tomographic scan analysis. *Int J Oral Maxillofac Implants* 17:854-860.

Veldkamp WJ, Joemai RM, van der Molen AJ & Geleijns J (2010) Development and validation of segmentation and interpolation techniques in sinograms for metal artifact suppression in CT. *Med Phys* 37:620-628.

Velloso GR, Vidigal GM Jr, de Freitas MM, Garcia de Brito OF, Manso MC &Groisman M (2006) Tridimensional analysis of maxillary sinus anatomy related to sinus lift procedure. *Implant Dent* 15:192-196.

Vercellotti T, De Paoli S & Nevins M (2001) The piezoelectric bony window osteotomy and sinus membrane elevation: introduction of a new technique for simplification of the sinus augmentation procedure. *Int J Periodontics Restorative Dent* 21:561-567.

Vercellotti T, Nevins ML, Kim DM, Nevins M, Wada K, Schenk RK & Fiorellini JP (2005) Osseous response following resective therapy with piezosurgery. *Int J Periodontics Restorative Dent* 25:543-549.

Verstreken K, Van Cleynenbreugel J, Marchal G, Naert I, Suetens P & van Steenberghe D (1996) Computer-assisted planning of oral implant surgery: a three-dimensional approach. *Int J Oral Maxillofac Implants* 11:806-810.

Vitkov L, Gellrich NC &Hannig M (2005) Sinus floor elevation via hydraulic detachment and elevation of the Schneiderian membrane. *Clin Oral Implants Res* 16:615-621.

Vlassis JM & Fugazzotto PA (1999) A classification system for sinus membrane perforations during augmentation procedures with options for repair. *J Periodontol* 70:692-699.

Wallace SS & Forum SJ (2003) Effect of maxillary sinus augmentation on the survival of endosseous dental implants. A systematic review. *Ann Periodontol* 8:328-343.

Wallace SS, Mazor Z, Froum SJ, Cho SC & Tarnow DP (2007) Schneiderian membrane perforation rate during sinus elevation using piezosurgery: clinical results of 100 consecutive cases. *Int J Periodontics Restorative Dent* 27:413-419.

Watzak G, Tepper G, Zechner W, Monov G, Busenlechner D & Watzek G (2005) Bony press-fit closure of oro-antral fistulas: a technique for pre-sinus lift repair and secondary closure. *J Oral Maxillofac Surg* 63:1288-1294.

Watzek G, Bernhart T & Ulm C (1997) Complications of sinus perforations and their management in endodontics. *Dent Clin North Am* 41:563-583.

Wendler D (1986) Nathanael Highmore (1613-1685) and the maxillary sinus. *Anat Anz* 162:375-380.

Whittaker JM, James RA, Lozada J, Cordova C & GaRey DJ (1989) Histological response and clinical evaluation of heterograft and allograft materials in the elevation of the maxillary sinus for the preparation of endosteal dental implant sites. Simultaneous sinus elevation and root form implantation: an eight-month autopsy report. *J Oral Implantol* 15:141-144.

Williams S (1996) Pearson's correlation coefficient. *N Z Med J* 109:38.

Wiltfang J, Schultze-Mosgau S, Merten HA, Kessler P, Ludwig A & Engelke W (2000) Endoscopic and ultrasonographic evaluation of the maxillary sinus after combined sinus floor augmentation and implant insertion. *Oral Surg Oral Med Oral Pathol Oral Radiol Endod* 89:288-291.

Wodak E (1961) Comparative temperature measurements in the maxillary sinus mucosa. *Monatsschr Ohrenheilkd Laryngorhinol* 95:278-282.

Woo I & Le BT (2004) Maxillary sinus floor elevation: review of anatomy and two techniques. *Implant Dent* 13:28-32.

Xie B, Yuan J, Zheng X, Wu Z, Wan J & Guo Y (2002)Measurement of ostium area of maxillary sinus on three-dimensional imaging. *Zhonghua Er Bi Yan Hou Ke Za Zhi* 37:38-40.

Xu M, Yang F, Wang RF (2011) Cone-beam CT analysis of human maxillary sinus: Anatomical considerations for sinus augmentation and implant insertion. *Shanghai Kou Qiang Yi Xue* 20:187-190.

Yang HM, Bae HE, Won SY, Hu KS, Song WC, Paik DJ & Kim HJ (2009) The buccofacial wall of maxillary sinus: an anatomical consideration for sinus augmentation. *Clin Implant Dent Relat Res* 11:e2-e6.

Zijderveld SA, van den Bergh JP, Schulten EA & ten Bruggenkate CM (2008) Anatomical and surgical findings and complications in 100 consecutive maxillary sinus floor elevation procedures. *J Oral Maxillofac Surg* 66:1426-1438.

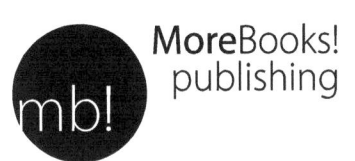

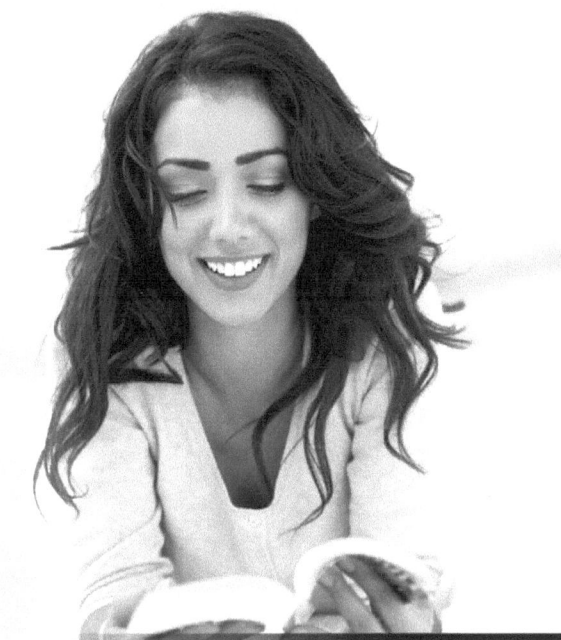

i want morebooks!

Buy your books fast and straightforward online - at one of world's fastest growing online book stores! Environmentally sound due to Print-on-Demand technologies.

Buy your books online at
www.get-morebooks.com

Kaufen Sie Ihre Bücher schnell und unkompliziert online – auf einer der am schnellsten wachsenden Buchhandelsplattformen weltweit! Dank Print-On-Demand umwelt- und ressourcenschonend produziert.

Bücher schneller online kaufen
www.morebooks.de

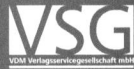

VDM Verlagsservicegesellschaft mbH
Heinrich-Böcking-Str. 6-8   Telefon: +49 681 3720 174   info@vdm-vsg.de
D - 66121 Saarbrücken   Telefax: +49 681 3720 1749   www.vdm-vsg.de

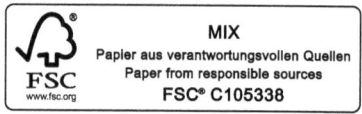

Printed by Books on Demand GmbH, Norderstedt / Germany